CW00665812

Clinical supervision
the principles and process

Copyright ©   Health Visitors' Association, 1995

published by
Health Visitors' Association
50 Southwark Street
London SE1 1UN

designed by
Peter Brawne

page make-up by
Quest, London EC1

printed by
College Hill Press Ltd. London SE1

ISBN   1 872278 29 9

Contents

Foreword [5]

Introduction [7]

Part one   **The principles of clinical supervision** [11]

1.1   History and background [11]

1.2   Defining clinical supervision [16]

1.3   Why clinical supervision? [20]

Part two   **The process of clinical supervision** [26]

2.1   Clinical supervision and language [27]

2.2   Clinical supervision and support [28]

2.3   Types of supervision [29]

2.4   Contracts and ground rules [31]

2.5   Content of supervision [32]

2.6   Frequency of supervision [32]

2.7   Time and place [33]

2.8   Confidentiality [34]

2.9   Codes of ethics and practice [34]

2.10   Recording sessions [36]

2.11   Interpersonal dynamics [37]

2.12   Wider contextual relationships [39]

2.13   Clinical supervision and management supervision [40]

2.14   The internal supervisor [42]

2.15   Training of supervisors [43]

Part three   **Issues for managers** [45]

3.1   Principles of good management practice [45]

3.2   Personal support [49]

Part four   **Models of clinical supervision in practice** [51]

Conclusion [78]

Appendices

I   The BAC code of ethics and practice for the supervision of counsellors [79]

II   Bibliography [85]

Acknowledgements

Grateful thanks are expressed to the following people for their very valuable contributions to this guidance document:

Mary Anthony; Mary Carter; Joan Heckels; Jackie Lawden; Anne McClelland; Helen Westbrook; Diana Roxburgh; Neil Brocklehurst; Jim Burden, Susan Mott; Angela Chapman; Chris Byrne; Sue Gregory; Helen Sudlow; Martin Ballard; Kathy Elloway; Gaynor Dixon; Nicci Cook; Catherine Jackson; Ralph Layland; Sue Botes; Margaret Buttigieg; Liz Day; Deborah Hennessy; Sue Jerram; Carole Dixon.

Special appreciation and thanks to the participants at the HVA regional workshops who contributed their definitions, and to the HVA members and members of the HVA managers sub-committee who provided the initial thinking on this subject.

A list of practitioners willing to be contacted on the subject of clinical supervision is available from the HVA.

Foreword

The challenge to the nursing profession set by *Visions for the future*,[1] to consider how it supports practitioners in their work by the introduction of clinical supervision, has led to much discussion and debate. In England, the nursing division of the department of health has itself funded two publications: one through the King's Fund;[2] the other through Manchester University.[3] In Wales, initiatives have taken place in the educational arena, with a course to help train supervisors now under way. Numerous trusts throughout the country are considering how clinical supervision can be introduced and maintained, and many models – some good, some less so – are emerging.

This publication from the Health Visitors' Association is a further contribution to the national debate. Its aim is both to stimulate further discussion and to promote advancement of practice in this important area.

It is written by an experienced health visitor, community nurse teacher and former senior NHS manager, who is also a qualified psychodynamic counsellor. It issues a number of thought-provoking challenges to practitioners and managers who are considering introducing clinical supervision: about their organisation and the management structure within it, and about why and how clinical supervision should be introduced.

Our aim in publishing this guidance is not to provide a single model for practice, nor to be prescriptive or directive about 'how to do' clinical supervision. Rather, the HVA's aim is to provide information to enable practitioners and managers out in the field to develop their own models, suitable for their place of work, and to offer a broad-brush framework of the key values and principles which can and should be considered when introducing clinical supervision.

Clinical supervision will only benefit the nursing and health visiting profession if it is seen as part of the fabric of the organisation. Management supervision and clinical supervision are different functions, and should not be undertaken by the same individual.

Their purposes are separate but complementary, and this must be recognised and understood by all within the organisation, from the chief executive to the practitioners in daily contact with the clients. It is only when the whole ethos of the organisation is one of the acceptance of the need for such staff support that clinical supervision can really be beneficial and aid the effective and efficient functioning of the organisation.

Although much work is presently being undertaken to introduce clinical supervision into nursing, there remains much still to be done. Its real benefit will be for those who follow us, as it becomes accepted as an essential part of working within the NHS.

I commend this publication to you. The need to promote the value of the contribution of nursing to health care has never been greater. Effective use of clinical supervision will play a major part in achieving this aim.

Margaret A Buttigieg
director
Health Visitors' Association

REFERENCES

1   Department of health. *A vision for the future: the nursing, midwifery and health visiting contribution to health care.* London: HMSO, 1993.

2   Kohner N. *Clinical supervision in practice.* London: King's Fund, 1994.

3   Butterworth C, Faugier J. *Clinical supervision: a position paper.* Manchester: Manchester University, 1994.

Introduction

It is to be welcomed that the nursing profession as a whole is beginning to look seriously at the issue of clinical supervision. It has long
been an established part of social work, counselling, psychotherapy
and psychoanalysis practice, and in the nursing specialties of mental
health nursing and midwifery. Its wider application to all nurses
and health visitors is timely, and long overdue.

The principle of clinical supervision is now an accepted part of
the national agenda for the development of the nursing, midwifery
and health visiting professions.[1] It is as though the 'search for health
needs' – that fundamental principle of health visiting[2] – by the
profession has revealed an unequivocal 'health need' within the profession itself for the kind of respectful, humane care we aim to
accord to our clients.

The present realities of increasing unemployment, homeless-
ness, poverty, and the poor health which goes hand-in-hand with
poverty[3] (an issue which the government's 'Health of the Nation'
white paper fails to acknowledge[4]); the inadequacy of resources to
provide effective care in the community;[5] all have an impact on the
individual nurse in the community, both professionally and personally. This, combined with the impact of the tremendous organisational changes brought in by the 1990 NHS reforms, the commercial
ethos of the internal market, and what many experience as an anti-
clinical and anti-clinician climate, adds to this stress, and carries
with it a de-valuing both of the clinician and the clinical work.

Implicit in all of this is a de-valuing of those whom the practitioner seeks to serve: the client and the wider community. Indeed,
the very concept of public service itself is increasingly seen as old-
fashioned and out of place. The values which influenced our commitment to the work, and our choice to follow the nursing profession, now seem to many to have little currency. In today's pres-
surised and under-resourced health services, many seem to have lost
sight of why they wished to do the work in the first place.

We entered the profession with a conscious sense of vocation:

a commitment to a public health service; a commitment to primary health care; a commitment to social justice. We shared the principles which underpinned the NHS when it was first introduced: the values of an equitable, universal, national health care service, funded through taxation and free at the point of delivery; a service which valued the individual and the community; a service which acknowledged their right to health care to meet – within realistic resource levels – their need for care; a service which respected their right to humane, respectful care and attention, and to protection from abuse and exploitation; the value of a trained body of professional midwives, nurses and health visitors, and of professional and adequately-resourced midwifery, nursing and health visiting services; the valuing of the individuals providing those services, through the provision of continuing professional education and development, and individual support to help them cope with the demands of their work.

These are the values which should shape our philosophy; principles which should underpin all our practice. 'Human services are the heart of our collective attempt to build a decent, fair, and humane society.'[6]

There is plentiful evidence to demonstrate that something more is necessary to help practitioners in their work. Increasing burn-out, absence and sickness rates;[7] the numbers of practitioners leaving the profession, all give strong indication that not enough is being done to prevent disillusionment, exhaustion and departure. The distress experienced by once dedicated nurses on reaching this state is hard for them to bear, and hard for their colleagues, who feel powerless to prevent it.

There are many examples of evidence that all has not been well for many years in the health and care services. Martin's shattering analysis of failures of care in UK long-stay hospitals, *Hospitals in trouble*,[8] asks the question: 'How is it that institutions established to care for the sick and helpless can have allowed them to be neglected, treated with callousness and even deliberate cruelty?' Martin's work is a careful examination of the findings of the major inquiries into long-stay hospitals. It makes salutary reading. Martin concludes: 'If there is a dominant theme which emerges it is the extent to which nurses experience anxiety... Managers will have to modify their roles to see themselves more as facilitators supporting and advising their staff in caring for individual patients.'

In the past decade there have been numerous major inquiries[9] into cases of child abuse, all of which have revealed what has amounted to a very serious failure of professional effectiveness. Among the significant findings, lack of supervision and of adequate support for clinicians have been highlighted as factors, and the need for specialist practitioners providing supervision in child protection work. Of particular significance is the Allitt inquiry.[10] This inquiry, as do the others, makes painful but necessary reading. But the whole document should be read, not simply the summary of recommendations. It is only in the detail of the whole document that the full impact of professional incompetence and lack of professional leadership and rigour can be fully absorbed, and the recommendations fully understood. Faced with the complete evidence, professional maturity demands that we acknowledge that Beverley Allitt was as much a victim as the innocent infants she killed.

Something more is clearly needed to help practitioners. This 'something more' must surely be dedicated attention to the needs of staff themselves: to their workloads, their professional practice and concerns and anxieties about it; to their 'feeling' state and their 'health' state; to their capacity for creative work, and its encouragement, and to establishing a place of safety where disappointment or failure in practice can be examined honestly, prejudices challenged constructively, and success and good work owned and applauded.

We speak and write of reflective practice,[11] yet experience out in the field suggests a very different reality. Time for reflection is, in fact, a rare commodity indeed. Clinical supervision provides just such a forum and space for reflection. That is why it is increasingly on our agenda. But it must not simply stay on the agenda, as a future luxury; it demands serious consideration, discussion and implementation now.

Clinical supervision will benefit the practitioner, their practice, and ultimately the client, be they individual, family, group or the wider community. The health service exists for the client; the client is our prime and primary concern. We should also remember that all of us working in the health service will ourselves be clients from time to time, and are potential clients all of the time. So too are our families, friends and loved ones. This thought may concentrate wonderfully the mind of any sceptics still doubting the need for clinical supervision.

The aim of this document is to provide health visitors and community nurses, their managers and professional development leaders, with a broad-brush framework of the values and principles of best practice which should underpin the implementation of clinical supervision. It does not set out to be prescriptive or directive; systems of clinical supervision must be flexible, and adapted to local circumstances and need. Its purpose is to be a starting point and source of reference, to spark, inform and guide discussion, to facilitate the development of systems of clinical supervision appropriate to the needs of practitioners and managers in the context of the community and primary health care services in which they work.

The terms 'health visitors and community nurses' will be used throughout the text generically to denote health visitors, school nurses, practice nurses, district nurses and other qualified nurses working in community and primary health care settings. References to 'managers' will also be relevant to team leaders and facilitators in primary health care. The term 'she' is used to denote both female and male practitioners. The 'client' may refer equally to an individual, family, group or community.

REFERENCES

1   NHSME. *A vision for the future: the nursing, midwifery and health visiting contribution to health care.* London: HMSO, 1993.
2   CETHV. *The principles of health visiting.* London: CETHV, 1977.
3   Wilkinson R, Quick A. *Income and health.* London: Socialist Health Association, 1991.
4   Department of health. *The health of the nation: a strategy for health in England.* London: HMSO, 1992.
5   Robinson R, Legrand J (eds). *Evaluating the NHS reforms.* London: King's Fund Institute, 1994.
6   Garner LH (jnr). *Leadership in human services.* San Francisco: Jossey & Bass, 1989.
7   Seccombe I, Buchan J. *Absent nurses: the costs and consequences.* Brighton: Institute of Manpower Studies, 1993.
8   Martin JP. *Hospitals in trouble.* Oxford: Blackwell, 1984.
9   Department of health. *Child abuse: a study of inquiry reports 1980-89.* London: HMSO, 1991.
10 Department of health. *The Allitt inquiry.* London: HMSO, 1994.
11 Burnard P. Improving through reflection. *Journal of District Nursing* 1991; 9, 11.

Part one   **The principles of clinical supervision**

I.I   **History and background**

Traditionally, the practice of clinical supervision has been associated
with Freud, with psychoanalytic training and practice, and with
psychotherapy. In these professions, as trainees reach the stage of
seeing two training patients two to three times a week or more,
they are expected to meet weekly with two separate supervisors; one
for each patient. Generally the patients will be of different genders.
This continues until the trainee qualifies, although many will continue with supervision after qualifying. Even the most experienced
of therapists will seek supervision of their own practice in some way
at times throughout their working lives.

In counselling, the practitioner is required both to have weekly
supervision during training, often in a group of fellow trainees, and
to remain in supervision following qualification for the rest of her
working life, as laid down by the BAC code of ethics for counsellors.[1]
A further stringent requirement is that the trainee in psychotherapeutic work will also be undergoing their own psychoanalysis or
psychotherapy, often in advance of as well as during training, and
usually for some time beyond qualifying. Each school of psychotherapy has its own regulations, but no reputable training establishment would countenance compromise on either of these requirements for supervision and therapy.

Being in supervision and being in therapy are not the same,
although the two are sometimes confused. In classical psychotherapy
training the supervisor does not and should not act as therapist to
the supervisee; nor does the therapist act as supervisor, although
there may be temptation to do so at times, and there can be 'grey
areas' where the roles overlap. The critical distinction is that clinical
supervision is to do with clinical practice, with the focus on the
patient or client; personal therapy focuses on the individual receiving therapy, and on their own inner and outer world.

Freud wrote[2] that the essential quality for the psychoanalyst is
'inherent insight into the human soul – first of all into the uncon-

scious layers of his own soul – and practical training'. Rollo May stresses[3] the importance of avoiding 'seeing others through one's own prejudices'; an 'ego bias (which) is clearly the worst stumbling block in the counsellor'. This principle can be held to apply not just to the trained counsellor but to all of us engaged in human services, not least in health visiting and community nursing.

In social work too, the tradition of supervision has long been established, usually for the individual practitioner. This is 'case' supervision, as distinct from managerial supervision or therapy. Such supervision begins in training and, again, is a continuing practice requirement.

Here in the UK social work as a profession developed largely as a response to social and material stress. In the USA the profession's beginnings were rooted more in psychiatry, and for this reason gave more primacy to the need for clinical supervision. Aware of this difference, in 1927 a group of social workers visited the USA, and in 1929 the first psychiatric social work training was established, at the London School of Economics. The training focused on the development of the relationship between practitioner and client as a tool for use in social work practice. As one experienced senior social worker, trained in the early 1960s at the LSE, puts it: 'In those days what we called "case work" then was much more what we would call counselling now. It was very individualistic and concentrated on the client's mental health and personal adjustment, and the supervision mirrored that. Now we are still concerned with the client as the focus, but the supervision addresses more issues of social justice for the client, and meeting the aims and objectives of the employing agency. Things have changed a lot. Counselling skills are still important though for the supervisor.'

The nursing profession can learn much from these other professional disciplines and their belief that clinical supervision is integral and essential to their work. It beggars belief that we have for so long failed to incorporate it as a defined component of practice. Any one of us looking back at the human pain and social distress of others to which we have been exposed – not to mention our own – must surely question what makes us suppose we can practise effectively without such a regular, conscientious examination of our work, of what might improve it and what impedes it, and of our own feelings about it.

There have been some developments in clinical supervision within the nursing profession as a whole: namely, in psychiatric nursing, and in midwifery where supervision and the role of the supervisor is formalised in a very specific way.[4]

As Simms relates[5] with respect to psychiatric nursing: 'In 1943 the Horder Committee recommended the development of supervision in practice. Opportunities for supervision to be integrated into mental health nursing education and practice were made more possible with the implementation of the 1982 Registered Mental Nurse syllabus. The holistic nature of this syllabus changed supervision from a concept into a reality, and to a more accepted way of working – not just for students, but for trained staff also. The practice of supervision in mental health nursing has gained momentum, as its value in helping to ensure safe and competent practice, and in developing the knowledge, skills, and attitudes of mental health nurses, has become increasingly recognised by the profession.'

However Carson[6] and others make the point: 'Although the concept of clinical supervision is well accepted in mental health nursing, it is less well established as a reality for most practitioners. It is clear that clinical supervision is certainly not yet the norm for the majority of mental health nurses; for the most part, the only form of clinical supervision to which nurses have access is provided by informal peer group support. There are of course notable exceptions where there has been an attempt to take the issue of clinical supervision seriously, but these examples are few and far between.'

This is even more the case for health visiting and community nursing. In health visiting and district nursing the supervision of post-registration students by specifically trained community practice teachers has been established for many years. With health visiting, as Twinn relates:[7] 'Clinical supervision occurs in two distinct phases: fieldwork practice and the period of supervised practice. These two components of the health visitor course were introduced following a revision of the curriculum in 1965 and have essentially remained unchanged since that time. Fieldwork practice provides students with an opportunity to rehearse health visiting practice in a protected environment under the guidance of an experienced practitioner who her/himself will have undertaken further education and training for this role'.

The main early influence on the development of formal standards for education and practice in district nursing has been the Queen's Nursing Institute (QNI). Founded in 1887, the QNI fostered 'a distinct "district nurse" culture...and part of that culture was the notion of proper supervision of individualised practice'.[8] In more recent years, the introduction by the UKCC of Project 2000 pre-registration nurse education, and of the PREP post-registration education reforms have brought into formal nursing currency the terms and practice of preceptorship and mentorship. These roles, and their relation to other supervisory and assessment functions, are summarised by Butterworth as:[9]

* 'mentor – an experienced professional nurturing and guiding the novitiate
* 'assessor – an experienced professional making judgements on another's ability to carry out procedures or interactions
* 'clinical supervision – an exchange between practising professionals to enable the development of professional skills
* 'preceptor – a teacher or instructor.'

The current climate in which community nurses struggle to practise effectively has generated much anxiety among practitioners about standards of practice and their ability to continue to provide services of quality. There is a sense of increased professional isolation; geographically from peers, and professionally from the dearth of senior nurse managers available to practitioners in all nursing specialties. This isolation makes it even more difficult to explore professional concerns and share anxieties, and thus increases both work pressure and personal stress. Repeated organisational changes tax even the most flexible of practitioners. Continuing clinical work while at the same time practising creatively through the development of imaginative ideas for future practice requires professional stability, boundaries and containment. Where these are available there may be less likelihood of adverse effects on clinical practice, the practitioner and the client, even in the midst of the kinds of upheavals experienced over the past 15 years; an issue which the department of health report into the 1994 health visiting market project makes clear.[10]

This fact seems now to have been recognised at national policy-making level. The department of health nursing division, in its 1993 strategy for the nursing profession,[11] included clinical supervision as an essential component in the development of health visiting, nursing and midwifery. In what can be seen as a clear policy directive for its development and implementation, target ten of *A vision for the future* states:[11] 'Discussion should be held at local and national level on the range and appropriateness of models of clinical supervision and a report made available to the professions by the end of the first year.' *Testing the vision*,[12] reporting progress so far on implementing the 'vision', found that discussions had been held on clinical supervision in 86 per cent of units, although the outcomes of these discussions, and whether they led to implementation of clinical supervision, was not reported.

The department of health has also supported two of the three texts we should see as essential reading on the subject of clinical supervision. These are:

- *Clinical supervision: a position paper*,[13] by professor Tony Butterworth and Jean Faugier of Manchester University; commissioned by the nursing division of the department of health and published in 1994
- *Clinical supervision and mentorship in nursing*,[9] published in 1992 and edited by the same authors
- *Clinical supervision in practice*,[14] also commissioned by the department of health nursing division, written by Nancy Kohner, and published by the King's Fund Centre nursing development unit in 1994. This text is complemented by a supplementary executive summary highlighting the issues for managers and health authority purchasers.[15]

REFERENCES

1   British Association of Counselling. *The code of ethics and practice for counsellors.* London: BAC, 1993.
2   Freud S. *A general introduction to psychoanalysis.* New York: Horace Liveright, 1920.
3   May R. *The art of counselling.* London: Souvenir Press, 1992.
4   UKCC. Midwives rules. London: UKCC, 1993.
5   Simms J. In: Wright H, Giddey M (eds). *Mental health nursing: from first principles to professional practice.* London: Chapman Hall, 1993.
6   Carson J, Fagin L, Ritter SA. *Stress and coping in mental health nursing.* London: Chapman Hall, 1995.
7   Twinn S. In: Butterworth T, Faugier J (eds). *Clinical supervision and mentorship in*

nursing. London: Chapman Hall, 1992.

8 Pateman B. In: Butterworth T, Faugier J (eds). *Clinical supervision and mentorship in nursing.* London: Chapman Hall, 1992.

9 Butterworth T, Faugier J (eds). *Clinical supervision and mentorship in nursing.* London: Chapman Hall, 1992.

10 NHS Executive. Health visitor marketing project. Project report. July, 1994.

11 NHSME. *A vision for the future: the nursing, midwifery and health visiting contribution to health care.* London: HMSO, 1993.

12 NHSME. *Testing the vision: a report on the progress in the first year of 'A vision for the future'.* London: HMSO, 1994.

13 Butterworth T, Faugier J. *Clinical supervision: a position paper.* Manchester: University of Manchester, 1994.

14 Kohner N. *Clinical supervision in practice.* London: King's Fund Centre, 1994.

15 Kohner N. *Clinical supervision: an executive summary.* London: King's Fund Centre, 1994.

1.2 Defining clinical supervision

In 1994, the HVA published a briefing document on clinical supervision, circulated to all its members through the *Health visitor* journal.[1] The paper usefully summarises the discussions about and definitions of clinical supervision, and sets out what the HVA believes to be the central principles and requirements for its implementation, including the following, succinct warning:

'Supervision has been an integral part of midwifery practice for a long time. The role, however, has not developed into one of empowerment or professional development; rather one of guidance and direction to ensure practice is correct. It is also used to discipline when practice goes wrong. One would not wish to see clinical supervision within nursing and health visiting develop in this way.'

The main point here would seem to be that the role of supervisor *vis à vis* health visiting and community nursing should not include the authority formally to discipline, direct or guide in a model of restrictive practice; rather it should be concerned with empowerment and professional development. This immediately raises other questions: what then would be its relationship to management, and – crucially and fundamentally – what precisely is clinical supervision?

A useful starting point is to state at the outset what it is not. As previously noted, it is not psychotherapy or counselling. This must be clearly understood. Nor is it directive management, individual performance review (IPR), or staff appraisal. It is not a form of disciplinary procedure; nor should it be used as a devious ploy to get rid of unwanted staff. It is not any of those many things which some nurses seem to fear it might be or could be used for.

Some of these widespread fears among practitioners are vividly expressed in comments from participants at workshops run by the HVA during its 1995 regional conferences. For example:

' ...it is not linked to a management role...'

' ...it should not be seen as threatening but enhancing the practitioner's awareness of issues'

' ...the relationship should be trusting, not threatening, and there should be mutual respect, empowerment of the individual and not control...'

' ...it is not a police inspectorate to be used by management...'

' ...it should not be threatening or destructive.'

That anxiety and misunderstandings exist is openly acknowledged in the literature. As Platt Koch has stated,[2] confusion about and resistance to clinical supervision could be 'depriving nurses of one of the most valuable tools in existence for learning and refining skills of assessment and treatment of patients'.

The same workshop participants also offered definitions of what they believed clinical supervision should be:

' ...the opportunity for one or more persons to discuss worries/problems around caseload management/child protection issues with a relevant senior professional, in order for that senior to provide support, to inform professional development and to monitor practice'

' ...the monitoring of clinical practice to maintain standards of care... (providing) support in stressful situations, but also on a regular basis, (preventing) stress and (promoting) sharing of knowledge'

' ...an opportunity to share clinical experience and knowledge and to measure personal standards against others...(concerned with) management, standards, individual personal development, education and support'

' ...a process which enables a practitioner to reflect on their practice using research in a constructive way...improving the quality of their work, relieving stress and isolation, and...supportive'

' ...a process of enabling a practitioner to reflect on their practice, identify what influences their practice, both positive and negative, and identify how a practitioner can learn from practice in order to become more effective'

' ...a formal process which is planned and programmed, which enables individuals and groups to develop their practice to meet the needs of clients'

' ...the opportunity to discuss and reflect on the processes in professional work with individuals and to consider how these affect the client and the worker and the effectiveness of the work.'

Interestingly, these comments also serve to indicate the essential elements many practitioners feel are missing from the current professional leadership and clinical development role.

The literature yields a number of definitions, some of which are quoted here. Hill[3] suggests: 'Supervision is a dynamic, inter-personally focused experience which promotes the development of therapeutic proficiency. One of the primary reasons for all supervision is to ensure that the quality of all therapeutic work with the client is of a consistently high standard in relation to the client's needs. Consequently, supervision must be acknowledged as a cornerstone of clinical practice.'

Here the emphasis is on quality and standards, and relates to the client's needs. The supervision encounter is alive and active, and one in which both supervisor and supervisee are equally engaged.

Hawkins and Shohet write:[4] 'Our experience is that supervision can be an important part of taking care of oneself, staying open to new learning, and an indispensable part of the helper's on-going self-development, self-awareness and commitment to learning.'

Here we are alerted to the importance of care of self, continuing self-development, self-awareness and the desire to go on learning. This readiness to continue with the learning suggests the importance of research to practice development.

Wright believes:[5] 'Supervision is a meeting between two or more people who have a declared interest in examining a piece of work. The work is presented and they will together think about what was happening and why, and what was done or said, and how it was handled, could it have been handled better or differently, and if so how?'

This underlines the need for a desire, opportunity and readiness to think about the work and to examine what else might have been done: honest scrutiny, in short.

Knapman and Morrison describe clinical supervision as:[6] '...a process in which one worker is given the responsibility to work with another to meet certain objectives. These objectives are competency, accountability, performance, on-going professional development and personal support.'

This definition is specific to child protection, and reminds us that we do have to meet certain objectives in our work; that we are professionally accountable, and that professional vigilance is required, particularly when working with vulnerable people.

The definition offered in the department of health strategy document *A vision for the future*[7] links supervision directly with the UKCC policy document *The scope of professional practice*.[8] The latter sets out the parameters for safe practice and educational requirements with respect to what is traditionally termed 'extended nursing practice'. In this context, *A vision for the future* states:[7]

'Clinical supervision is a term used to describe a formal process of professional support and learning which enables individual practitioners to develop knowledge and competence, assume responsibility for their own practice and enhance consumer protection and the safety of care in complex clinical situations. It is central to the process of learning and to the expansion of the scope of practice and should be seen as a means of encouraging self-assessment and analytical and reflective skills.'

The HVA briefing document[1] reminds us that the aim of *The scope of professional practice* was 'to encourage nurses, midwives and health visitors to take accountability and responsibility for their own practice and the education required for that practice', and that the department of health withdrew its guidance delineating the 'extended role' of the nurse following its publication.

Taken together, these various definitions describe a process which is essentially positive; one which not only respects the client's needs but also demonstrates a profound respect for the value of nursing practice, and for the practitioner herself. There is, in short, nothing to fear from clinical supervision. On the contrary, there is much to be gained from a process the prime aim of which is to restore the centrality of professional clinical practice to the health service. It makes clear that the work of the clinician should be taken seriously, and examined with stringency by the practitioner with another (or others), in a climate of compassion.

REFERENCES

1   HVA professional briefing. Clinical supervision. *Health visitor* 1995; 68, 1: 28-31.
2   Platt Koch LA. Clinical supervision for psychiatric nurses. *Journal of Psychological Nursing* 1986; 26, 1: 7-15.
3   Hill J. Supervision in the caring professions: a literature review. *Community Psychiatric Nursing Journal* 1989; 9,5: 9-15.
4   Hawkins P, Shohet R. *Supervision in the helping professions.* Milton Keynes: Open University Press, 1989.
5   Wright S. In Butterworth T, Faugier J. *Clinical supervision and mentorship in nursing.* London: Chapman Hall, 1992.
6   Knapman J, Morrison T. The benefits of supervision. *Primary Health Care* 1994; 4, 6: 21-22.
7   NHSME. *A vision for the future: the nursing, midwifery and health visiting contribution to health care.* London: HMSO, 1993.
8   UKCC. *The scope of professional practice.* London: UKCC, 1992.

1.3 Why clinical supervision?

Clinical supervision is necessary – essential, indeed – primarily because of its focus on the client and the protection of the client's interests and rights. In this respect, it could be said to be one aspect of patient advocacy.

The emphasis is on actual clinical practice, discussed in a regular and systematic way. Such a process is not currently widely available within health visiting and community nursing. This is not to say that no attempts are ever made to examine or reflect on practice; simply that the reality of current constraints and demands militates against them. Intentions are sound, but external reality reduces good intentions to *ad hoc* opportunities, with both participants aware of the time constraints on the other. Last minute cancellations, sudden summonses to supposedly crucial meetings, the nightmare of finding mutually convenient diary space, and the increasing use of the mobile phone all lead to a way of working that is simply reactive. This itself raises fundamental questions about how we manage time.

The implementation of regular clinical supervision could go a long way to redress this imbalance. In a reputable psychotherapeutic training establishment, and for reputable practitioners, missing or cancelling supervision is regarded very seriously indeed. The trainee or practitioner's obligation to the client requires attendance at supervision. Equally, the supervisor has a similar obligation to the client, through the trainee or practitioner, which demands a similar commitment. Clinical supervision is embedded as a priority within the professional culture; only pre-arranged breaks, illness, bereavement or emergency are accepted as valid reasons for cancelling. Other important matters will be planned around the supervision session.

1.3.1   **Reflective practice**

Regular clinical supervision provides the space and opportunity to reflect on practice: why the work is being approached in a particular way; what might be difficult; the nature of the interaction with the client; whether the philosophy and principles of health visiting are underpinning practice, and if they can be demonstrated. The health visitor or community nurse gives an account of her practice in what is essentially a benign and sympathetic environment. This should facilitate an enhancing of professional and personal self-confidence, which in turn will facilitate the leadership role which should be there for every practitioners to both use and develop.

Leadership is extremely important, and increasingly so in today's flattened organisational structures and fragmentation of service provision. As Garner writes:[1] 'Leadership need not be a rare skill – leaders can be developed; leaders need not be charismatic and leadership need not be manipulative or exist only at the top of the organisation. Especially in human services, leadership should pervade an organisation. Commitments to clients, service, employees, and the public – not manipulation – is the crucial element of this theory.'

1.3.2   **Developing practice**

At national political level, and percolating down throughout the health service, the emphasis is on outcomes and efficiency and cost. As playwright Dennis Potter once said in another context:[2] 'Everything was given, in a sense, its price tag, and the price tag became the only gospel and that gospel in the end is a very thin gruel indeed, and if you start measuring humankind in those terms, everything else then becomes secondary...'

Of course, outcomes, efficiency, and the sound investment of funds are important, but they are also 'very thin gruel indeed' if process, quality and effectiveness are ignored. Clinical supervision has to acknowledge all these factors.

The first principle of clinical supervision must be that clients should benefit, individually and corporately, directly and indirectly. Effective supervision should assist the development of professional practice, of the profession as a whole, and of organisations. It should provide the opportunity to further the integration of theory and practice; to increase awareness of research findings, and to encourage the practitioner herself to become a 'searcher' after more effective ways of working. As Ekstein and Wallerstein point out:[3] 'If supervision is used as a method of unfolding the best capacities... one which will not destroy (her) initiative and (her) curiosity...it will have contributed to the creation of a research atmosphere.'

A theoretical underpinning to practice is undeniably important. So too is an established knowledge-base of certain facts, and the accessing of information. As Casement observes,[4] we need to be mindful that 'theory helps to moderate the helplessness of not-knowing. But it remains important that this should be servant to the work...and not its master... By listening too readily to accepted theories, and to what they lead the practitioner to expect, it is easy to become deaf to the unexpected'.

The text from which this comment comes refers to psychotherapy, but serves as a reminder to both supervisee and supervisor of the importance of keeping an open mind in the work; that the client may not fit easily into accepted theory, and we should not attempt to force her to do so. 'Becoming deaf to the unexpected' is something that no health visitor and community nurse can afford to do. An environment in which clinical supervision is accepted as a fundamental part of professional practice will render this less likely.

Nevertheless, if we are to have the confidence to treat theories as 'servant', and to be able to put them on one side when the situation demands it, we need first to know and understand them, in order to give ourselves the choice of whether to apply them in practice.

In her discussion of the gap between theory and practice, Twinn[5] describes how integration of the two for students may be 'influenced by the (community practice teacher's) interpretation of professional practice'. This, she believes, 'may be restricted to a narrow range of practice skills, or encompass the much broader definition of professional practice which includes the intuition in practice by which practitioners make sense of the unique practice setting'.

Clinical supervision offers the opportunity for vision to be widened; for the practitioner to take a broader view of professional practice, and to apply her own skills and knowledge gained from experience to a given situation.

1.3.3 Defensive practice

By offering a 'facilitating environment',[6] clinical supervision should contribute to a lessening of professional anxiety. Systems of defence against anxiety built up by staff groups can substantially affect organisations; practitioners may develop their own ways of working to protect themselves against unmanageable anxiety; ways of working which may seem to offer some personal benefit but which do not benefit the client. These defences are usually unconscious and strongly held.[7] This is less likely to occur in an organisation where staff are encouraged on a regular basis to discuss their practice and explore their feelings and anxieties about their work. The 'holding' experienced in the supervision should enable painful areas of the work to be examined. A less defended and appropriately supported workforce will have a positive impact on service provision and on the client. This is an important point for chief executives and health services purchasers to understand, and a critical part of the role of the nurses on NHS trust and health authority boards is to facilitate such understanding.

1.3.4 Maintaining standards

From 1 April 1995 every nurse, midwife and health visitor must meet certain statutory requirements in order to renew her registration every three years. These requirements are laid down in the UKCC's post-registration education and practice (PREP) regulations.[8] The main requirements, which apply to every individual registered nurse, midwife and health visitor, are that she should:

* undertake at least five days of study activity in the three-year registration period. This study must be relevant to her professional registration and role
* complete a notification of practice form
* maintain an ongoing record of her personal professional develop-

ment (which may be subject to audit).

The UKCC describes the primary purpose of these post-registration requirements to be to 'contribute to the maintenance and development of professional knowledge and competence'.[8] The UKCC further states that 'the UKCC register is an instrument of public protection. It is the only means by which an employer or a member of the public can check reliably that you do have the necessary qualifications for the delivery of safe and effective midwifery and nursing care'.[9]

Clinical supervision is inextricably linked with this. Its purpose, like that of PREP, is to improve standards of patient and client care, both directly and indirectly. In this context, the UKCC states of PREP: 'When the new system is fully in place, being registered with the UKCC will have a much greater meaning for you and other practitioners in terms of professional standards. In future, your UKCC registration will not only mean that you have reached the necessary professional and academic standards for initial registration, but that also you have, on a three-yearly basis, maintained and developed those standards through additional learning activities for the benefit of patient and client care'.[9]

Using the process of clinical supervision will inevitably contribute to the maintenance and development of professional standards and indicate which learning activities would be particularly beneficial to the practitioner for client care. Clinical supervision will also promote self-appraisal and examination of practice, and the development of what Casement calls 'the internal supervisor.'[4]

Specifically with reference to clinical supervision, the guidance fact sheets issued by UKCC to explain the PREP requirements[9] suggest that the planning of professional development, implementation of the personal action plan, and self-appraisal for personal profiling may be usefully discussed with the manager, supervisor of midwives, clinical supervisor, tutor or a colleague. Thus implicit in the UKCC's standards for maintaining and developing professional skills and knowledge is the acknowledgement of the role of the clinical supervisor, and the full expectation that clinical supervision will become a reality in professional, clinical practice.

REFERENCES

1   Garner LH (jnr). *Leadership in human services.* San Francisco: Jossey Bass, 1989.
2   Potter D. *Seeing the blossom: two interviews and a lecture.* London: Faber and Faber, 1994.
3   Ekstein R, Wallerstein R. *The teaching and learning of psychotherapy.* New York: International Universities Press, 1972.
4   Casement P. *On learning from the patient.* London: Routledge, 1994.
5   Twinn S. In: Butterworth T, Faugier J (eds). *Clinical supervision and mentorship in nursing.* London: Chapman Hall, 1992.
6   Winnicott D. *The maturation process and the facilitating environment.* London: Karnac, 1990.
7   Menzies Lyth I. *Containing anxiety in institutions. Selected essays volume one.* London: Free Association Books, 1988.
8   UKCC. *The future of professional practice: the council's standards for education and practice following registration.* London: UKCC, 1994.
9   UKCC. *PREP and you.* London: UKCC, 1995.

Part two   **The process of clinical supervision**

A key text when planning the implementation of clinical supervision is *Supervision in the helping professions.*[1] This, while not concentrating on any specific profession, touches all. Hawkins and Shohet stress 'the need to integrate both the emotional and the rational, the personal and the organisational, and the educative, supportive and managerial aspects of supervision'. They go on to state that 'this integration inevitably provides a creative tension that has to be constantly understood and worked with'. This is the process which should be achieved through the supervisory relationship.

In the introduction to this guidance reference was made to the conscious sense of vocation among those who choose to enter the nursing professions. What, though, of our unconscious motives for choosing this work? How much has it to do with meeting our own needs? Is it a desire to make reparation, perhaps; a sense of guilt; a need to be needed? Each of us will have some underlying motivation. This does not in any way negate our work, nor render invalid our conscious commitment. Nor does it give us licence to offer a 'wild analysis' of the motives of our colleagues, but there are distinct advantages in having a self-understanding which helps us to be honest with ourselves, within ourselves; honest in the work and our reactions to it.

Hawkins and Shohet emphasis this, and all health visitors and community nurses, wherever they are working in the organisation, should read their work, particularly in the climate of today's NHS.

Hawkins and Shohet make reference to the 'wounded helper'; a theme which is also found in Nouen's *The wounded healer.*[2] Our own vulnerability can be one of our strongest assets, if we can acknowledge it to ourselves – and even, with courage, to others. It enables us to recognise ourselves in others: in the client, the supervisee or supervisor, the manager, the GP, the chief executive.

Vulnerability is not found in the client alone, however much better such a thought might make us feel. Vulnerability is in us all, and acknowledging this will help towards true equity and partnership.

Guggenbuhl Craig, in *Power in the helping professions,*[3] reminds us how our very zeal to help can be unhelpful. Our 'helpfulness' is likely to be more genuine, appropriate and client-centred if moderated by self understanding.

REFERENCES

1   Hawkins P, Shohet R. *Supervision in the helping professions.* Milton Keynes: Open University Press, 1989.

2   Novens H. *The wounded healer: ministry in contemporary society.* London: Darton, Longman & Todd, 1994.

3   Guggenbuhl Craig A. *Power in the helping professions.* Dallas: Spring Publications, 1971.

2.1   Clinical supervision and language

Some of the terminology of clinical supervision has been a cause of nervousness and suspicion. Given the culture of nursing, its hierarchical history, and the current style of defensive and macho management, this is hardly surprising. Words like 'supervision', 'rigour',' 'discipline', 'monitoring', 'contracts' and 'control' have become imbued with negativity. Many nurses have moved into the community precisely to escape the oppressiveness of the traditional, hierarchical hospital setting, and to be able to work more 'independently'. Community nurses derive great pride from describing themselves as 'independent and autonomous practitioners in our own right'. Further, a distortion has occurred which makes it increasingly difficult for us to use language in an honest and truthful way. There is, it would seem, such a climate of fear and oppression within the NHS that any move towards critical examination of practice is regarded with suspicion.

However it has to be stated that the concept of 'the independent practitioner in our own right' is a myth, and untrue. We work interdependently, with our colleagues and with our clients. Our 'right' to practise exists only by virtue of government statute, and we are required to abide by certain rules and regulations, and by our code of professional conduct. If we fail to meet the standards expected of us, we can be censured by our own professional regulatory body and prevented from practising. This serves to protect both the public and the practitioner.

The difficulty arises when the assumption is made that clinical supervision is intended to seek out and censure poor practice: that is, a defensive process, rather than one which seeks to develop practice; a process that is concerned with telling rather than listening on the part of the supervisor, and with direction rather than enablement. In fact, the converse is true; but for staff to believe and experience this is not easy, and requires radical change within the nursing culture.

As stated previously, there is nothing to fear from clinical supervision. We need not be afraid that clinical practice or the role of the practitioner will in any way be marginalised by the clinical supervision process; indeed, both will be enhanced. But it can be painful, and sometimes frightening, to expose our work to the scrutiny of others. Questions of judgement, criticism and censure inevitably arise: 'Have I got it right?'; 'Will I get into trouble?' Dr Mildred Pott, a child psychiatrist teaching health visitor students in the 1960s and 1970s, advised one student: 'With reverence risk all'. Adam[2] refers to 'fears that do not allow (us) to venture'. To go forward, we have to take risks.

Equally, we need feedback on the positive aspects of our work. We need to have our good practice affirmed, as well as reflecting on what we might do better. Every one of us worries to some degree about what other people (professional colleagues or others) think of us. However, as self-confidence grows and we learn to be more open, we find we mind less about this. The supervisory relationship in the context of clinical supervision offers us this opportunity.

REFERENCES

1   Butterworth T, Faugier J (eds). *Clinical supervision and mentorship in nursing.* London: Chapman Hall, 1992.
2   Adam D. *The open gate.* London: Triangle/SPCK, 1994.

2.2 Clinical supervision and support

The whole issue of staff support to health visitors and community nurses, and nurses in general, is one of crucial importance. It has to be admitted that the profession as a whole has been notoriously bad at supporting staff, and nurses are often reluctant to request support, believing it unreasonable to want or even express the need for it. Self-care does not feature highly on many nurses' agendas. The long hours and unpaid over-time that many community nurses work; the snatched meals and missed meal breaks; the continuing availability via the telephone, crammed diaries, cancelled holidays and contact with work during holidays all confirm this self-neglect.

Put simply, if we do not care for ourselves, we cannot care for others; if we cannot look after ourselves, we cannot look after others; if we do not respect ourselves, we cannot respect others. We know this, but too often we fail to address it. Nurses work on relentlessly while experiencing enormous personal tragedy, and colleagues collude.

Clinical supervision will not solve this problem. It is very important to state this. Clinical supervision does not replace the need for staff support groups and for staff counselling services. Nor does it replace the need for courteous, sensitive, consultative organisational management. All these require attention, and never more than now, but they are distinct from clinical supervision.

Clinical supervision and staff support must both be provided, separately and alongside individual staff development programmes, if health visitors and community nurses are to be enabled to work healthily, effectively and creatively.

That said, a support element is intrinsic to the clinical supervision process. This, while not 'cosy', should be holding; while not counselling in a formal sense, will be listening to the individual's 'feeling state' as she carries out her work, and will use counselling skills; while not occupational health, will take note of the supervisee's 'health' state.

2.3 **Types of supervision**

Supervision can be provided in a variety of ways.

1   *One-to-one supervision.* One supervisor provides clinical supervision for one practitioner. This is the common practice for qualified counsellors. It allows the supervisee professional intimacy and a real space, place and dedicated time, unthreatened by demands from peers (sibling rivalry). How this relationship is experienced by both participants will be crucial to the supervision process, and may need to be discussed from time to time.

2   *Group supervision with a specified supervisor.* One supervisor provides clinical supervision for a group of, say, three supervisees.

Usually two of the three will present in the session, while the third listens and observes but can take 'emergency time' to speak if needed. The sessions are usually rotated, so that the supervisees know in advance who is to present their work. Sometimes all three may present, with the supervisor leaving it to the supervisees to determine how much time each needs. Again, there are no hard-and-fast rules; the group will decide for itself how the time is apportioned and managed. How they do this, and how they relate to each other and to the supervisor, will be of interest to the supervisor.

3   *Peer group supervision.* Three or more practitioners of equal status act as supervisors of each other's practice, in the context of a group. This could be seen as the least expensive (most cost-effective) form of supervision. However some would see it as informal supervision; others simply as support. It has a potential inherent weakness in that it can allow a perpetuation of practice which, in other supervision models, might be explored more rigorously.

Yet other alternative forms of supervision, summarised by Houston,[1] are:

* one-to-one peer supervision, in which roles are alternated
* one-to-one sessions where the supervisor is from another discipline
* group supervision in a 'hybrid' mix of disciplines, and
* network supervision.

These various alternatives and their appropriateness to the particular clinical setting could be discussed at the consultation stage. Such discussions would address the mix of community nurses within a team and the particular configurations which might be most beneficial and challenging. Some of the configurations may contribute better than others to team-building and team-working.

No hard-and-fast rules can be laid down as to how the clinical supervisor is chosen. However experience in the field would suggest that it is helpful when the supervisee can choose her clinical supervisor. There are considerable advantages in this approach, and clearly it would be totally inappropriate, and unlikely to achieve positive outcomes, if a supervisor who was not acceptable were to be imposed on a practitioner. No supervisor should be prepared to accept such a position (see also section 2.9).

It should also be born in mind that a formal qualification in, say, community practice teaching does not necessarily qualify an individual to take the role of clinical supervisor (see section 2.15 on training of supervisors).

REFERENCE

1   Houston G. *Supervision and counselling.* London: Rochester Foundation, 1990.

2.4   Contracts and ground rules

The practical guidelines in Kohner's work[1] offer an invaluable framework for the development of local systems of supervision, and should be read in full. With respect to the supervisory relationship, the guidelines state:

● 'The content of supervision should be carefully defined, with boundaries agreed about what is and is not to be dealt with in supervision time. The processes to be used should also be made clear,' and

● 'The relationship between supervisor and supervisee should be formally constituted. Ground rules should be negotiated and agreed.'

Any discussion of supervision has to consider both the supervisee and the supervisor. The contract and the ground rules will have to address the following issues:

● confidentiality

● whether there are, or should be, any links with management (for example, performance appraisal)

● frequency

● location

● time management

● record keeping, and

● (in terms of content) boundaries and framework.

There needs to be an awareness of the dynamics of supervision: issues such as parallel processes, transference and countertransference, the appropriate use of counselling skills and avoidance of 'quasi-counselling', and matters of ethics. More detailed exploration of these issues can be found in section 2.11.

REFERENCE

1   Kohner N. *Clinical supervision in practice.* London: King's Fund Centre, 1994.

2.5   **Content of supervision**

The content of supervision should be agreed in advance between supervisor and supervisee:

* what should be brought to the session; what would not be considered appropriate

* whether and how the agenda is set, with the recognition that the supervisee will initiate those matters to be included.

These boundaries will be fluid. For example, the supervisor may offer, subject to the agreement of the supervisee, to concentrate in a subsequent session on an issue which has arisen in the current session, or the supervisee may make a specific request to do so.

The allocated time may be used in a number of ways, as agreed by supervisor and supervisee. The session may be educative, reflective and exploratory. Organisational issues may arise and require discussion, not in a managerial sense, but in terms of how an issue raised in the supervisory process can be managed or incorporated in practice, or an examination of the difficulties to which it may give rise in practice. If either participant feels that a particular issue or topic constitutes a 'boundary break', this should be raised and explored. The ability to be assertive as well as reflective is crucial for both participants.

2.6   **Frequency of supervision**

Frequency of supervision is a vexed question. In health visiting and community nursing, ideally supervision should take place weekly to four weekly. Any less frequent timetabling would be unsatisfactory, for all the following reasons.

1   The process and practice of supervision is based on a relationship and, as in every relationship, this develops over time and has to be worked at.

2   Health visitors and community nurses daily face complex and often harrowing situations, whether working with child protection, families of concern or people who are dying or bereaved. That, very probably, colleagues have 'coped' without clinical supervision for years is no reason to expect them to continue to do so. What has this 'coping' cost the individual practitioner in emotional terms? What has been the cost to the service and the client in terms of impeded professional development? These are the crucial questions

which must be asked.

3   Given the number of families and clients with whom health visitors
and community nurses are working, any period longer than four
weeks makes it difficult to examine any aspect of the work in
depth. A predictable response will be: 'Where will the time come
from?' It will come from time that is currently lost through sickness
and absence from burn-out. The time is already there; it must be
re-allocated, better managed, reclaimed. This is not an impractical
suggestion; it can be achieved, if we really want to use our time
more effectively.

The length of the supervisory session again varies. Ideally it will
be 50 minutes for individual supervision, and one-and-a-half to two
hours for group supervision. An inability to find this time, and to
make any necessary changes to working patterns in order to accommodate it, suggests organisational or individual resistance, and
needs to be examined very honestly.

2.7   **Time and place**

Location, day and time of supervision sessions should be fixed and
regular, with work planned around this professional commitment.
Supervision, as previously stated, should not take second place to
other commitments. Supervision should be seen to have equal status with other work priorities; other meetings will not be deemed
'more important'.

Ideally, supervision sessions should take place in a pleasant environment, in the same room, booked on a regular basis. A cupboard
space or a table in a corridor are not acceptable. The session should
be free from all intrusions: from other people, telephone calls,
requests for 'vital' pieces of information, or 'vital' messages.
Supervision should be seen as time dedicated to the supervisee, and
should be respected. These boundaries of time and space should be
kept. Herein is both discipline and support.

Timing is important. The session should begin and end
promptly. This means appropriate planning ahead on the part both
of supervisor and supervisee; commitments on either side of the
supervision session should not be allowed to encroach. It may be
difficult to resist the prevailing culture in the health service, in
which cancellation, leaving early, or arriving late from a previous

engagement which has carried over to deal with an unexpected, urgent matter are common practice. A recent, increasingly intrusive phenomenon is the mobile phone. We have to learn to resist these diversions and distractions, and to be more assertive. The adherence to boundaries of time can be a helpful discipline in other parts of working life, and can have a positive influence within the working unit as a whole.

This must be spelled out. Care-less use of time leaves us disabled and dis-eased. We need to use our abilities with ease, and careful management of time will assist us in this.

2.8 Confidentiality

It is important that confidentiality is discussed at the preparatory stage, when negotiating and agreeing the contract and establishing the ground rules. What can remain confidential, and where the boundary to confidentiality comes to an end, must be clearly understood and agreed by both parties. Matters should only be taken outside the context of supervision with the agreement of both parties, and it should be agreed who should do the taking, where, and to whom.

The supervisor needs to be able to recognise within herself what is motivating her wish to make a boundary break. Is it clearly imperative that the matter be taken elsewhere, or is it a response to the supervisor's own difficulty in holding the supervisee through a complex situation? This is an area which requires much thought and debate, within the profession and in training workshops. Managing this kind of dilemma will depend much on the supervisor's own self-awareness and understanding, and on her personal and professional integrity. This is a place where her ability to stand equi-distant between the organisation, the supervisee and the client will be tested.

2.9 Codes of ethics and practice

As registered nurses, both supervisee and supervisor will, of course, be bound by the UKCC professional code of conduct, which seeks to safeguard the interests of the patient and client and to protect the practitioner. However the codes of ethics and practice drawn up by the British Association of Counselling will also offer useful guidance and reference in the planning, negotiation and implementation of clinical supervision, and in governing its ongoing practice.' The BAC has published codes of ethics covering a number of aspects of the counselling process: on the use of counselling skills, on counselling practice, and on the trainer/trainee student counsellor relationship. Most pertinent to this guidance is the BAC code of ethics and practice for the supervision of counsellors. This will be particularly useful to units embarking on the introduction of clinical supervision, and is therefore reproduced in full at Appendix 1.

Trusts and units are recommended to draw up their own code of ethics and practice (or protocol), using the BAC code as a basis.

The BAC code of ethics covers the nature of supervision; issues of responsibility, and issues of competence. The code of practice deals with management of supervision work, and confidentiality.

Most supervisors of counselling are in private practice (as are many of their supervisees), but the BAC code applies equally to practitioners employed in an organisation or agency. It addresses a number of issues of particular anxiety to health visitors and community nurses and, with the exception of the question of payment of fees to the supervisor, all parts can be applied in principle to supervisors working in NHS units and trusts. The code does not conflict with the UKCC professional code of conduct, or other UKCC guidance, and is applicable to all types of supervision.

The BAC code of ethics and practice for the supervision of counsellors states: 'Ethical standards comprise such values as integrity, competence, confidentiality and responsibility.' It establishes principles of respect and confidentiality not only with respect to the client but also to the practitioner. It reminds supervisors that any necessary discussion with colleagues of an individual practitioner 'should be purposeful and not trivialising'. This is something we should all strive towards, at all times and in all contexts, whether discussing clients or colleagues.

Also addressed in the code of practice is the critical issue of breakdown in the supervisory relationship. The supervisor may feel she is unable adequately to fulfil her role towards the supervisee; the supervisee may feel she is not receiving the supportive guidance she needs. Section C 2.13 of the BAC code of practice states: 'Where personal disagreements cannot be resolved by discussion between supervisor and (supervisee), the supervisor should consult with a fellow professional and, if appropriate, offer to refer the (supervisee) to another supervisor.'

These arrangements may not apply easily to the NHS organisational context, particularly in rural, isolated areas where there may be few practitioners suitably qualified and prepared to act as supervisors. A formal process must be agreed whereby the supervisor or supervisee (or both) can seek third party intervention in resolving the breakdown of the supervisory relationship. In the context of NHS organisational structures, the supervisor might discuss the situation (with the knowledge of the supervisee) with a peer who is also fulfilling the supervisory role, and arrange to refer the supervisee to another supervisor. The supervisee might similarly talk with another supervisor, and seek referral elsewhere. In the absence of such a third party, a line manager, professional development officer or senior nurse might fulfill this role.

The primary aim should be, where at all possible, to resolve the situation through discussion, mediated where necessary by the third party. However, where the situation has totally broken down and cannot be resolved, alternative arrangements should be made. Where there is no alternative source of supervision within the relevant discipline in that locality, it may be necessary to go outside the health visiting or community nursing profession. Alternative sources of supervision might come from the fields of mental health nursing, social work, or possibly clinical psychology.

Organisations must make every effort to ensure there is access to an alternative source of supervision. Line managers and senior nurses should be sympathetic and receptive to expressions of concern or complaint from staff. Unsatisfactory clinical supervision may be more damaging to the individuals involved than absence of supervision altogether.

REFERENCE

1   British Association of Counsellors. *The code of ethics and practice for the supervision of counsellors.* London: BAC, 1988.

2.10   **Recording sessions**

How the sessions are recorded, where these records are kept, and who (if anyone outside the supervisory relationship) has access to them are very important matters which must be negotiated and agreed in advance between the supervisor and supervisee.

A joint record of the key points raised and discussed during each session, and any conclusions or decisions reached, will provide a useful source of information, both as an *aide memoire* for application to the practice setting, and to maintain continuity if a topic or situation arises again or is returned to. The joint record should be completed at the end of each session.

Both participants may wish to make their own, personal notes during the session. These may then be used to inform the agreed, joint record, but should not be seen as a formal record of the session. The supervisee will also find it useful to record details from the supervision session in her personal professional profile, both as a store of pointers for practice development and as a record of the professional development process itself in terms of creative thinking and reflective practice.

This joint record (and any personal notes if kept) should be completely confidential to the supervisor and supervisee, unless both parties agree to share them with a third party. The joint record (and any personal notes) should not be kept with the supervisee's employment files. Applying the empowerment principle of the parent-held child health record,[1] it could be argued that the supervisee should hold this joint record, so that she can refer to it as needed and include it as a dynamic part of her professional development process.

Full names of any clients discussed should not be recorded on any of these records, as a matter of confidentiality.

REFERENCE

1   HVA. *In their own hands: introducing personal (parent-held) child health records.* London: HVA, 1991.

2.11   **Interpersonal dynamics**
The health visitor, school nurse, practice nurse and district nurse all work with people, on a daily basis. All their clinical work involves relating to another individual, or to individuals within a group or community, and the working day will always include some contact with another, be they client or patient or colleague. In the ebb and flow of the interpersonal encounter, things happen between us: in

the use of words, in our gestures, in our thinking and in our feeling. We sometimes know when our thoughts and feelings do not accord; when our words do not match our thoughts or feelings. People affect us in different ways, as we affect other people. Sometimes we understand why we react as we do; at other times we do not. Our unconscious is strong, but as our conscious understanding increases, so too does our self-awareness and our self-understanding. The more we understand ourselves and accept ourselves, the easier it is to understand and accept other people. The more aware we are of our own faults and failings, the less likely we are to allow prejudices and assumptions to create a stumbling block in our clinical practice and in our relations with clients, colleagues and others.

The supervisee and supervisor are also in a relationship. Simms cites Proctor:[1] 'Overall the quality of the supervision depends on both parties' abilities to communicate clearly and openly. The development of this ability is the foundation of... learning and is the stuff of counselling and interpersonal practice. It pre-supposes a high degree of self-awareness, interpersonal sensitivity and political nous.' It is this capacity, our readiness to risk self-disclosure about the 'feeling state' in our work, that is germaine to a good supervisory relationship. This requires a climate of trust.

Helpful also is an understanding of the processes of transference and countertransference which are experienced between the supervisee and supervisor, and between the client and the supervisee as practitioner. Perry[2] describes these processes:'The space between people is rapidly filled with projections. Both (nurse) and client project onto each other. These projections distort the space between them, thus making it difficult for them to relate to each other. Such distortion is called transference and is mirrored by counter-transference.'

Greenson's definition, cited in Perry,[2] is also helpful: 'It is the experiencing of feelings, drives, attitudes, fantasies and defences towards a person in the present which do not befit that person but are a repetition of reactions originating in regard to significant persons in early childhood, unconsciously displaced onto figures in the present.' Perry[2] also reminds us of Jung's comment: 'The transference itself is a perfectly natural phenomenon which does not by any means happen only in the consulting room – it can be seen everywhere.' Balint[3] describes countertransference as the whole of our responses to the client or patient, including our feelings and behaviour and attitudes.

Views and theories on these matters vary widely; what matters is that we are aware of our own 'feeling state' in the work. Such awareness is helpful because of what is called the 'parallel process'. Millar writes, in a different context but adapted here:[4] 'Research has shown that a parallel process of interpersonal dynamics operates in supervision. The interaction between the practitioner and the client is reflected in a similar way in the interaction between the supervisor and (the supervisee). Thus the (supervisee's) problems with the supervisor are related to the client's problems with the (practitioner) and vice versa. It is crucial that the supervisor be aware of this process, and be prepared to interpret and work through the problems and possibilities which arise because of it.'

This does not have to be so heavily used as some may fear, but an awareness that it happens can be useful, and can serve as a tool in the practice setting. Langs[5] usefully elaborates on the unconscious communication between the supervisee and supervisor.

These are all subject areas which should be on the supervision training agenda.

REFERENCES

1 Simms J. In Wright H, Giddey M. *Mental health nursing: from first principles to professional practice.* London: Chapman Hall, 1993.
2 Perry C. *Listen to the voice within.* London: SPCK, 1991.
3 Cited by Kohon G (ed). *The British school of psychoanalysis: the independent tradition.* London: Free Association Books, 1986.
4 Millar J. *A dictionary of pastoral care.* London: SPCK, 1990.
5 Langs R. *Doing supervision and being supervised.* London: Karnac, 1994.

2.12 Wider contextual relationships

While the relationship between the supervisor and supervisee(s) is key, there are other relationships within the organisational and practice contexts which must be taken into account.

Ekstein and Wallerstein's work[1] offers useful guidance on this issue. Described by Millar[2] as 'the classic reference book in the field of supervision', this fascinating read provides an in-depth exploration of the process of supervision. The authors refer to what they term the 'clinical rhombus': that is, the necessary relationship that exists between administrators, supervisor, practitioner and client. The book examines the conflicts that may arise over issues of training, research, organisational administration and clinical work. Similar tensions exist, as we know, within the health service, and in the complexities which have to be managed. Millar writes:[2] 'In supervision, the supervisor stands at the centre of a triangle which involves the needs and demands of a) the agency... b) ...the practitioner, and c) the client. The supervisor must have the requisite relationship skills to understand, and stay equi-distant from, the needs of the agency, the practitioner, and the client.'

In today's health service, the supervisor is required to have an understanding of the needs both of the provider and the purchaser, and of the nurse and client.

REFERENCES

1   Ekstein R, Wallerstein R. *The teaching and learning of psychotherapy.* New York: International Universities Press, 1958.
2   Millar J. *A dictionary of pastoral care.* London: SPCK, 1990.

2.13   **Clinical supervision and management supervision**
A fundamental principle of clinical supervision is that it should be distinct and separate from management supervision. The two must not be confused. To combine the roles is likely to interfere with the process of clinical supervision, consciously or unconsciously. It would undermine the environment of confidentiality and trust, and undermine the principle of honest disclosure, sharing and discussion, and the development it aims to achieve. It is for this reason that the line manager should never undertake the role of supervisor to those staff for whom she holds management or disciplinary responsibilities. Any moves to establish links between clinical supervision and the formal disciplinary process should be challenged.

This is not to say the two should never touch. Clinical supervision is integral to good management, which in turn is integral to an effective, healthy organisation.

In the process of reflective practice, some issues will, and should, arise from clinical supervision – notably, professional development and training needs – which may require management support and funding. Managers should be kept informed of the contribution of supervision to staff performance, and to service and individual staff development. They will wish to know that it is taking place, and that it is achieving positive outcomes; we will wish them to know it is making a positive contribution to the organisation as a whole. It would be unreasonable to expect managers to acknowledge the need for clinical supervision, which may require considerable organisational change, and then render it so sacred that nothing may be known of it.

What must be avoided is the misapplication of clinical supervision in the formal disciplinary process. Indeed, maintaining this critical separation may help avoid situations where disciplinary action is needed. Errors of omission or commission can frequently be traced back to a neglect of the professional, clinical or personal needs of the individual practitioner for supportive guidance and counselling. This may be a point when a contribution from the clinical supervisor, with the agreement of the supervisee, can save a situation degenerating into a matter of formal censure or dismissal.

To maintain the clarity of this separation, formal systems of communication between the clinical supervision process and organisational and line management should be discussed and agreed in the planning stage, and set down in the protocol or code of practice.

A joint report on the supervision process, based on the joint record kept by the supervisor and supervisee, could be supplied to management as an annual appraisal and assessment. However such a report should not be incorporated in or used as part of any disciplinary process, nor in performance appraisal for the purpose of determining pay and grading levels.

Reports could be written separately by the supervisor and supervisee and then amalgamated, or the report written jointly. Any report to management must be agreed between the participants.

This joint report might cover the following areas:

- development of clinical skills
- development of reflective practice skills
- development of caseload management ability
- development of inter-personal skills (with clients/colleagues/the organisation)

* development of presentation skills
* development of leadership skills
* awareness of ethical issues
* management of boundaries with clients and with the organisation
* evidence of ability to apply theory and research to clinical practice
* identification of areas of strength and weakness
* evidence of ability to learn from the supervision process
* evidence of ability to analyse and learn from practice setting
* ability to learn from colleagues' presentations, and apply to practice
* identification of areas of practice needing development/training
* areas in which development/training achieved
* positive achievements in the past year
* goals/hoped-for achievements for the coming year.

These are suggestions only; issues for inclusion should be agreed between supervisor and supervisee, and will vary according to the individual practice setting.

2.14 **The internal supervisor**

The internal supervisor is emphasised in the work of Patrick Casement, which is also useful and relevant to clinical supervision in the health visiting and community nursing contexts.

Casement writes:[1] 'At the outset, (students) naturally rely a good deal upon the advice and comments offered by the supervisor. With time, these supervisory insights should become more integrated into the on-going work with a patient.' He continues: 'During the course of being supervised, therapists need to acquire their own capacity for spontaneous reflection within the session, alongside the internalised supervisor. They can thus learn to watch themselves as well as the patient, now using this island of intellectual contemplation as the mental space within which the internal supervisor can begin to operate.'

Jacobs[2] observes: 'Supervision...moves the process of supervision of a single example of work...to a continuous internalised supervision of oneself and of one's skills and ability to understand the client.'

These descriptions mirror the concept of reflective practice and the process of 'learning through practice', as described by Schon,[3] and by Fish, Twinn and Purr.[4]

The ability to stand apart internally, both from self and from the client, while still in the process of interacting with the client is important. It should not be confused with standing aloof, 'not getting involved', or denying feelings; this would severely damage clinical practice.

We can use this self-awareness of our inner responses to the client and to the situation to improve and develop our work. Indeed, it is this very use of self in our work that makes clinical supervision essential.

REFERENCES

1   Casement P. *On learning from the patient.* London: Routledge, 1994.
2   Jacobs M. *Psychodynamic counselling in action.* London: Sage Publications, 1988.
3   Schon D. *Educating the reflective practitioner.* San Francisco: Jossey Bass, 1987.
4   Fish D, Twinn S, Purr B. *How to enable learning through professional practice.* London: West London Press, 1989.

2.15   **Training of supervisors**

It is important that all would-be supervisors receive training, as well as receiving clinical supervision themselves as they practise. Training needs will vary according to the requirements of the individual practitioner. However all preparation for the role must include the following basic requirements:

● counselling skills, particularly in skills of active listening and responding, and accurate reflecting[1]

● an understanding of the importance of the supervision framework and the need to respect boundaries, and

● an understanding of interpersonal dynamics, including both transference and countertransference[2] and the parallel process.

Some understanding of the theories of Donald Winnicott[4] in relation to mothers and their infants such as 'mirroring' and the 'good enough mother' may be helpful in considering the facilitating environment in which supervision can take place. Mirroring describes the process whereby the experience of the supervisee is reflected back, rather than the agenda of the supervisor forcing the pace;[3] being 'good enough' does not require perfection, but enough 'holding and containment' to provide appropriate security for confidence and trust to be established. At the same time supervision should be of sufficient 'ordinariness' to discourage idealisation of the supervisor, and should encourage and facilitate the development and growth of the supervisee.

All supervisors would benefit from an understanding of group dynamics, but this is particularly important for those supervisors engaged in group supervision.[5, 6]

REFERENCES

1   Jacobs M. *Swift to hear: facilitating skills in listening and responding.* London: SPCK, 1985.
2   Jacobs M. *Still small voice: an introduction to pastoral counselling.* London: SPCK, 1993.
3   Winnicott DW. *Playing and reality.* London: Routledge, 1991.
4   Winnicott DW. *Maturational processes and the facilitating environment.* London: Routledge, 1991.
5   Bion WR. *Experiences in groups.* London: Routledge, 1989.
6   De Board R. *The psychoanalysis of organisations.* London: Routledge, 1978.

Considerable emphasis has been placed on the possible anxiety of
the practitioner at the prospect of the implementation of clinical
supervision, and how it may be used or misused. But what of the
anxieties that managers may have? These are likely to include practical and organisational issues such as implementation, cost, staff
time, implications for purchaser contracts, job descriptions, who
should do the supervising, supervision training, and the specific
requirements of GP fundholders. They are likely too, to be concerned about the distinction between clinical supervision and
management supervision.

Some managers may feel clinical supervision poses a possible
threat to their management role. Perhaps, like the practitioner, they
may fear loss of autonomy, of power, of authority. We should not
deceive ourselves; power, authority and the opportunity to influence as managers are heady potions, particularly for those to whom
they are rarely granted. We would not seek them out, or accept
them when offered if we didn't want them, whatever our outward
protestations. Having got them, it can be very difficult to let them
go, or to have them taken away, as many nurse managers side-lined
by organisational change will know.

As previously stated, a critical consideration is whether line
managers should act as clinical supervisor to the community nursing staff for whom they are responsible. This is not recommended
as good practice. The potential for the blurring of distinctions
between supervision and control, and between critical appraisal and
discipline, could seriously undermine the climate of trust, honesty
and partnership integral to the effective supervision process.

3.1   **Principles of good management practice**
The principles of health visiting,[1] and their underlying philosophy
and values, again offer a useful framework within which to discuss
implications of clinical supervision for managers, and the role and
responsibilities they should take on.

The principles – the search for health needs; the stimulation of awareness of health needs; the influence of policies affecting health, and the facilitation of health-enhancing activities – should underpin the practice of the community nurse manager in her relationship to the community of health visitors, district nurses, school nurses and/or practice nurses for whom she is responsible. In this way 'health needs' will be seen to encompass personal as well as professional, emotional as well as physical health; the health status of the practitioner will be seen as a determinant factor influencing her effectiveness in her contribution to the health status of the client. Thus the commitment of managers to ensuring clinical supervision is made available must surely be unequivocal. If not, the nurse manager should perhaps ask herself, why not?

1   *The search for health needs of staff*, to enable them to offer an effective service, requires the manager to listen to what community nurses are saying; at times, more importantly, to what they are not saying. Much of it may already be known, but it is important to find the time to listen, and to address what is being heard.

This is not easy. The job of the health service manager is no sinecure. It can pose enormous difficulties, challenges and, for some, dilemmas of conscience when personal as well as professional values feel under threat. Many managers are only too aware of the stress and constraints with which community nurses struggle, but are unable to make dedicated time available to offer the individual support required, because of other demands. However, the provision of regular clinical supervision for her staff can also assist the manager, by freeing her from the anxiety and guilt she may feel in not being able to offer this as part of her management role. This, in itself, can further assist her in letting go of the defensive management practices which so often accompany anxiety born out of the burden of responsibility. This freeing up and letting go can allow the manager herself to be more flexible, creative and innovative, and to further her development as a leader.

Garner cites the Bennis and Nanus analysis of leaders,[2] where they make a critical distinction between managers and leaders: managers 'do things right', they suggest; leaders, however, 'do the right things, are visionaries, change the metabolism of their organi-

sations, introduce new ideas, policies, and methods to suit changing times, (and) articulate vision'.

They go on to state that: 'Leaders articulate a vision that provides focus and infuse daily activity with meaning. By communicat-
ing that vision to others they build trust in their vision by building
an organisation that can provide accountability, predictability and
reliability. They live their vision themselves and lead by example.'

Consulting with community nurses, listening to their views and
anxieties concerning their professional 'health' needs, and to their
responses to and ideas about clinical supervision, will assist in
pointing the way forward. As Kohner observes:[3] 'All staff should be
involved in the process of planning and introducing a system of
clinical supervision.'

2   *Stimulating an awareness of health needs* requires the manager to
bring to the attention of as many colleagues, in as many forums as
possible, the arguments for clinical supervision as a necessary component of good practice, and to stress the anticipated benefits to
the practitioner, the client, the service, and the organisation.
Raising this 'awareness' should also extend to the potential purchaser, be they health authority or GP fundholder. Where this is
achieved, no purchaser would consider contracting services where
clinical supervision was not an integral part of the organisation.

The role of the nurse working in the purchasing authority is
equally crucial here. The absence of such a nurse will make still
more crucial the ability of the community nurse manager to influence and persuade managers of (market, if you will) the necessity of
clinical supervision. It should be enough simply to state that supervision is good in itself, and essential for good practice. However
where such arguments cut no ice, a reminder of the tragedies that
have occurred, the subsequent public inquiries, and their recommendations, should be used to demonstrate the need. Clinical
supervision is proactive as well as reflective.

3   *The influence of policies affecting health* includes such matters as:
●   the place accorded to clinical supervision by the trust/employing
authority
●   its place in the business plan

● its inclusion in job descriptions and contracts of employment, which would include not only willingness to accept supervision, but also to train as supervisors

● a strategy and time scales for the incremental implementation of clinical supervision across the whole range of health visiting and community nursing services.

Equally important will be its inclusion in service contracts agreed with the purchasing authority, and the consequent cost implications. The short-term cost implications will arise from consultation and negotiating time, and the training of supervisors. In the long-term however, it should prove a highly cost-effective professional practice. Clinical supervision should bring positive benefits to standards of practice; to the practitioner and the client; to the service, and to the community as a whole. The policies influenced by the manager should therefore include monitoring, evaluation and measurement to test this hypothesis.

The department of health, despite endorsing – indeed, initiating – the impetus towards clinical supervision, has made clear there will be no extra funding. The money has to come out of existing resources. It has earlier been suggested that additional funding is not necessary; that time and resources can be found in the reduced sickness and absence levels and improved staff morale generated by a more benign cultural climate within the health care organisation; by better time-management, and by replacing reactive management and clinical practice with proactive practice. This hypothesis would also need testing.

Particular negotiation will be required with respect to practice nurses employed by general practitioners, and to community nursing services purchased by GP fundholders. Model five in the final section of this guidance (p.62) suggests how this may be achieved through establishing links with trust managers and human resources departments.

4 *The facilitation of health-enhancing activities* will include the provision of training for supervisors; the necessary linking with the human resources department, and the encouragement of those staff with training in counselling skills and practice to participate in some way in both the teaching and learning of supervision.

The key health-enhancing activity will be the provision of the clinical supervision itself. An overall health-enhancing activity will be the involvement of staff at each stage in decisions about the framework and format of the clinical supervision: namely the type of supervision, its frequency, who will be supervising whom, the form it will take (mixed or intra-disciplinary), and the content of supervision training.

• Managers will also have to address any ongoing professional and individual development needs of staff raised through the clinical supervision process.

3.2 **Personal support**

Another area in which the manager should take a lead is the additional support required for staff: that is, the provision of staff counselling services as a necessary part of the employing organisation. However, the lack of support and frequent self-neglect rife within the nursing profession apply equally to managers, at all levels. Jaundiced staff may laugh at the picture of the executive nurse going home to weep, but it does happen. Dehumanising and demonising our colleagues makes it easier to blame them, and to use them as scapegoats.

Managers need to ensure their own support, and this may have to be found outside their immediate unit of organisation. A useful example of the benefits of this, both for the individual and the organisation, is offered by the experience of one senior manager, a health visitor, who sought on-going professional support outside the service while managing an organisation recovering from a sad history and great pain. She wished to be able to be fully available to the staff and to the organisation, but not at the expense of her own self and values. She wrote:[4] 'The unconscious is amazing. Staff, not knowing I was in analysis, came to ask me if I would support their seeking clinical supervision of their own specialty, in this instance music therapy, and nurses requested the time for their own professional counselling to enable them to work more effectively with their clients and their staff. All of which, of course, I whole-heartedly endorsed and encouraged. The art therapist remarked that in her specialty she felt that the patients and clients could sense a difference in the climate of the service.'

The manager's potential for influencing and achieving change in participation and collaboration with staff can be very considerable. Self-care assists in the care of others.

REFERENCES

1   CETHV. *The principles of health visiting*. London: CETHV, 1977.
2   Garner LH (Jnr). *Leadership in human services*. San Francisco: Jossey Bass, 1989.
3   Kohner N. *Clinical supervision in practice*. London: King's Fund Centre, 1994.
4   Fletcher W. Unpublished papers. 1982-1989.

Part four   **Models of clinical supervision in practice**

That there is interest in addressing clinical supervision in many
parts of the county is evident. The King's Fund Kohner publication[1] presents five case studies, including one from the community
– the Stepney neighbourhood nursing team. The department of
health is funding 18 evaluation projects, which include seven community sites.[2]

This section offers ten examples of models of clinical supervision currently operating in health visiting and community and
practice nursing, in various sites and units. The sample is not scien-
tifically selected, and includes both successful and less successful
examples of approaches adopted. The aim is to offer a usefully critical perspective on current initiatives to put some form of clinical
supervision into practice.

There are similarities between the various models, and some
considerable differences. The differences are to be found particularly in frequency; whether or not there is a contract; managerial
involvement; recording of sessions; training for supervisors, and
supervision for supervisors. It is interesting to note that in one
model use of the terms 'supervisor' and 'supervisee' is explicitly
avoided, as it is seen to 'feed into' a hierarchical structure.

A consensus among all those contributing to this section, both
from recently qualified practitioners and experienced senior clinical
staff, is that clinical supervision has made a difference: a difference
in confidence and openness. Other differences – specifically in relation to practice – await further evaluation. We can only hypothesise
that a more confident and open health visitor or community nurse
is going to make a more effective contribution to community
health care services for her client.

The models are described under uniform headings, in the words
of the individual(s) contributing their experiences.

Model one   **From the perspective of the clinical manager/supervisor**

1   **Length of time clinical supervision has been implemented**
Three months. By the end of the year all nurses in the trust are
expected to be in receipt of clinical supervision.

2   **Nursing specialties involved**
All health visitors and district nurses.

3   **How clinical supervision is practised**
Peer supervision on a one-to-one basis, using Proctor's 'formative,
restorative, normative' model.[3] Concerned with reflecting on practice, exploring the work, and developing plans.

4   **Frequency and length of sessions**
Monthly, for one hour. The supervisor records the planning, which
is initiated by the supervisee. A record is made of what happens in
the session, and of the action plans. The supervisor signs the record
and the supervisee keeps it. It is their (the supervisee's) property.
Documentation and files have been specially designed for clinical
supervision.

5   **Links with individual performance review**
The supervisee would themselves take personal development issues
to IPR. The fact that the staff members were engaged in clinical
supervision would be noted, and if they were not this would be
seen as significant.

6   **Contract between supervisor and supervisee**
The contract is signed in advance of commencing clinical supervision. This is written into the ground rules.

7   **Training for supervisor**
Three full days, exploring concept and practice of clinical supervision, reflective practice, reflecting back, and raising awareness.

8 **Supervision for supervisor**
Each supervisor is supervised by a peer.

9 **Monitoring**
There is a form for staff to complete to indicate how long they have been in supervision.

10 **Evaluation**
A research and development officer will do the evaluating. S/he will be requesting feedback from staff.

11 **Audit**
Not yet, although there is a peer audit of documentation owned by supervisees.

12 **Impact of clinical supervision**
We have realised there are a whole lot of issues to be addressed. Recently a very experienced health visitor was describing how helpful she finds clinical supervision.

13 **Place in business plan**
Yes, it is seen as important. Training needs have to be highlighted, and these have to be made clear in the contracts.

14 **Special staff support services**
There has been approval at trust board level for a counselling service for staff. It is envisaged that people already on the staff who are trained in counselling will provide that service. We have a 'health at work' group that considers staff health needs.

There is a supervision support group for supervisors, and a clinical practitioners' support group run by a senior nurse clinical practitioner.

15 **Additional comment**
Everyone should receive clinical supervision as a part of their role. It should not be an option. There is pain as well as advantages, but this needs to be worked through. This stage has been achieved through a concerted effort.

Model two   **From the perspective of the clinical specialist**

1   **Length of time clinical supervision has been implemented**
We have spent four to six months in consultation and discussion and raising awareness among staff. We obtained training for ourselves, and attended the HVA course. From this we learned that time would be well-spent meeting with staff initially in groups to learn their worries, discuss the benefits of clinical supervision, and encourage supervision to be practitioner-led.

We have two models: individual supervision, which has been taking place for six months, and group supervision, which has been happening for four months.

2   **Nursing specialties involved**
Health visiting at the moment.

3   **How clinical supervision is practised**
a   Individual supervision is practitioner-led. The health visitor requests the supervision session. They know that we are available. This started on a child protection model. There is a review date set and so it becomes rather like a rolling programme. You might see someone every three months. Some practitioners you see a lot; others not. It depends on the issue.
b   Group supervision consists of a group of five or six health visitors, meeting every four to six weeks. After six months the cycle will be reviewed and evaluated. Really, it is monthly supervision. The people who meet are from a defined geographical patch, and are a mixed group. The group is facilitated by a clinical nurse specialist. One or two members will bring an issue – usually clinical work but it can be anything from transfer of records to problems with a new family. People learn from each other. Each practitioner is encouraged to write her own reflective diary after the session.

4   **Frequency and length of sessions**
Individual: as requested. Group: monthly, for sessions of between one and a half to two hours.

5   **Recording sessions**
    The group members keep their own reflective diaries; the clinical
    nurse specialist also keeps a reflective diary.

    In individual supervision there is a simple form for completion.
    We record the name of the health visitor, the date of session, the
    issue/discussion, and the action plan. Both sign it and both retain a
    copy. The health visitor may keep her notes with the appropriate
    family notes, or at her work base. The clinical nurse specialist keeps
    her copy in a separate file, to which only she has access. We also
    record review date and when the action plan is to be achieved. We
    haven't decided how long to keep these yet. There is no manage-
    ment involvement in this, and this is very helpful.

6   **Links with individual performance review**
    None, and no IPR at the moment.

7   **Contract between supervisor and supervisee**
    This is established at the very beginning and can be written down if
    the supervisee wants. It sets out the supervision process, agreed in
    consultation with the group. The group negotiates the venue, sets
    the framework and so forth.

8   **Training of supervisor**
    Clinical supervision is in our job description, and the nurse educa-
    tion adviser in the trust has a remit to ensure advice and training
    for clinical supervision is established. There have been a number of
    in-house sessions, and we are fortunate in that there is a good net-
    work of people where clinical supervision is already in place, espe-
    cially with community psychiatric nurses and learning disability
    nurses. There is the opportunity to learn from them, how they do
    it, the pitfalls, the mistakes. The HVA training course was very use-
    ful indeed. We looked at the development model of supervision:[4]
    supporting, informing, being a catalyst and being challenging.
    There was an opportunity to look at different models: experiential
    learning and a non-directive approach. We looked at the relation-
    ship between the supervisee and the supervisor, and the roles and
    responsibilities of both. We also have someone who has been under-
    taking a national board diploma module on clinical supervision.

9 **Supervision for supervisor**
I receive supervision from within the trust, from someone with a psychiatric and education background with supervision skills. My supervisor is not a health visitor. We meet monthly for one and a half hours, at set dates and times. I have a written contract which includes the frequency, time and the date of six sessions, with a seventh for review and evaluation. I initiate the agenda.

10 **Monitoring**
Not yet; too early.

11 **Evaluation**
We hope that the reflective diaries which the health visitors are asked to keep will assist us in this. We are working on a standard for clinical supervision.

12 **Audit**
Not yet. The nurse adviser for the trust has used a questionnaire to see where we are at, and this will be redone in six months.

13 **Impact of clinical supervision**
The difference is somehow tangible; there is a sense of more openness and a positive approach.

14 **Place in business plan**
Not known.

15 **Special staff support services**
In one area there is a health visitor staff support group, which meets monthly. There is a counselling service available for practitioners, and staff support each other.

16 **Additional comment**
There are three clinical nurse specialists for health visitors, and one has recently been appointed for school nursing, so clinical supervision will be developed with the school nurses. In six months things may be different, and we will know more. Everyone will develop their own model. With respect to GP fundholding, we are looking

at a model in one specific practice for clinical supervision for all the nurses in the primary health care team.

We have had a lot of support. It is important not to rush into clinical supervision; to take time, to read, to consult and negotiate. What is so good is having permission, having the time to do it.

Model three   **From the perspective of the informal supervisor**

1   **Length of time clinical supervision has been implemented**
I have been used as a source of informal supervision since I moved from my last post two years ago. This was part academic, part research, and concerned with reflective practice.

2   **Nursing specialties involved**
Health visitors, school nurses.

3   **How clinical supervision is practised**
In the main in the service it is authoritative, and defensive, and concerned with complicated cases and court evidence, and with children on the register. Procedures are checked and it seems to be fear-dominated; a defensive practice for management rather than for practitioners. It is fear-dominated, through fear of comeback. It is not into the affective domain for practitioners at all. I offer informal supervision to those who approach me for it, and often in new development posts. We look at different models of working and how to deal with other people in a bureaucratic structure, and how to deal with those who are tied into ways of working which are more procedural and akin to policing.

4   **Frequency and length of sessions**
Ad hoc.

5   **Recording sessions**
The supervisee is advised to keep a record for their own personal development. The supervisor keeps notes which are seen by the supervisee, and these are kept filed at the supervisor's home.

6 **Links with individual performance review**
None through the supervisor. The supervisee is advised to raise at her IPR any developmental needs which have been highlighted through the informal supervision process. This has proved to be very effective.

7 **Contract between supervisor and supervisee**
The supervisee understands there will be no miracles. The supervisor wants to know why she has been approached and for what purpose. Critical support is offered, but it is up to the supervisee to solve problems. The supervisor undertakes to be a resource in helping her, and will attempt to offer a balanced view.

8 **Training for supervisor**
No formal training. Supervisor has run courses on reflective practice, linked with research post, and is used to working in collaborative way with people as equals. It became easier to be honest with people – colleagues and clients.

9 **Supervision for supervisor**
Uses colleagues, on an informal basis. Could work without, but the work is challenging and difficult and there is a need to check it out.

10 **Monitoring**
None.

11 **Evaluation**
The supervisee and supervisor decide together whether it is worth continuing. If the supervisor decides it is inappropriate for any particular matter, she will indicate who the appropriate supervisor might be.

12 **Audit**
None for informal supervision.

13 **Impact of clinical supervision**
The practitioner is more confident and assertive; begins to decide objectives; begins to see goals and progress. It is easy to think noth-

ing has happened, as often the milestones reached are only small. However sickness rates have been seen to drop while in supervision, and to rise for one recently-qualified practitioner when supervision had to stop.

14   **Place in business plan**
Not known. The contract specifications contained vague, commercial jargon.

15   **Special staff support services**
There were staff support groups. People are reluctant to seek support. An active HVA branch helps.

16   **Additional comment**
There are two sorts of clinical supervision: one collaborative, the other authoritative. The word 'supervision' implies a hierarchy. The culture is hierarchical and punitive. To have the line manager as supervisor makes for difficulty, and clinical supervision should be disassociated from line management.

Clinical supervision would make such a difference. It should be part of ongoing training work. Some of the best tips I've learned have been from other practitioners. I like the opportunity to give something back.

Practitioners really need clinical supervision, but real change takes time; we cannot expect changes over-night. Change has to be nurtured, and the whole process must be seen through.

Model four   **Peer group supervision**

1   **Length of time clinical supervision has been implemented**
Three to four months, as a pilot scheme. The pilot will be evaluated after six months.

2   **Nursing specialties involved**
The pilot scheme includes health visitors. It is envisaged that eventually all district nurses and community psychiatric nurses will receive supervision.

3   **How clinical supervision is practised**

This is essentially peer group supervision. It can be used within a speciality, or with nurses within the primary health care team, or within a nursing unit. One has already been started which includes practice nurses, district nurses, the midwife, the health visitor and the social worker, at her own request. We also hope to include a new CPN.

At the moment we cannot be too specific about how it will all work out. The pilot scheme consists of a group of 12-13 health visitors within a locality. We meet at a specific time, every other Monday, for a one and a half hour session. Using a 'round table' approach, one of us acts as co-ordinator on a three-month rota.

We use the Proctor model.[3] Our approach is not very structured, however. It is more about education and support. The managerial part is about self-management; how we move our practice forward. We discuss ideas and clinical practice in general, but not individual cases yet.

We look at how we work, and share ideas. I suppose we are slightly task-orientated. It needs to be more supportive and a smaller group may help here. Perhaps three people working with child protection issues may find this less threatening than a large group. We have to take care not to be judgemental, and to learn how to react to each other.

4   **Frequency and length of sessions**

Alternate weeks for one and a half hours.

5   **Recording sessions**

No records are made. We agree a list of issues we want to discuss, and the rota of co-ordinators.

6   **Links with individual performance review**

None. We do not have IPR within the trust; nor is it to be introduced. The clinical supervision will make us look at our own developmental needs and encourage us to introduce some plan of action.

7   **Contract between supervisor and supervisee**

None.

8 **Training for supervisor**
   We do not use the terms 'supervisor' and 'supervisee' as these seem
   to indicate a hierarchical structure, which we do not have within the
   trust at all. A multidisciplinary working party consisting of health visitors, district nurses and community psychiatric nurses has been involved in setting up afternoon workshops on clinical supervision. We
   look at where it comes from, the work of Faugier and Butterworth,[5]
   and at appropriate research, and people go away and think about it.
      No-one is under any duress to attend, but most people do.
   We've tended to concentrate on the positive aspects rather than
   negative ones.

9 **Supervision for supervisor**
   Not relevant.

10 **Monitoring**
   We have built in an on-going evaluation of the pilot scheme, and
   will feed back at the end of the six month pilot period.

11 **Evaluation**
   See above. We may also look at the knowledge and attitudes people
   had prior to the onset of the pilot scheme and at the end of it.

12 **Audit**
   Not yet.

13 **Impact of clinical supervision**
   So far people are very keen. It seems to have drawn people together
   in a positive way, and provides a focus for meetings. Health visitors
   seem to be incorporating this into their work and are more positive.
   We seem to be more confident in managing ourselves; more
   autonomous, and more confident in making our own decisions and
   not asking management so much. We seem to be able to move forward ourselves. One manager is responsible for 280 staff, so clinical
   supervision is going to be very important.

14 **Place in business plan**
   Not written down.

15 **Special staff support services**
None. The trust buys in personnel services from another trust. They are good and will act promptly. Occupation health services are shared with the acute trust. We have four locality managers, and if there is a stressful difficulty they are the first point of contact.

16 **Additional comment**
We have a very non-hierarchical organisation, and we are very much influenced by the approach of the director of nursing services, who trusts us and tells us so. He is not eager for us to promote a supervision system which involves much form-filling, or has a hierarchical aspect to it. The trust is successful and has achieved several star ratings. People are expected to manage themselves.

Model five **Developing a model for practice nurses**

1 **Nursing specialties involved**
Practice nurses.

2 **How clinical supervision is practised**
There could be a variety of developmental models to accommodate different levels of experience. It is important to take into account the development of the individual practice nurses.

3 **Frequency and length of sessions**
Minimum of once every four weeks; 45 minutes to one and a half hours, depending on whether group supervision or one-to-one. Supervision is carried out in the context of a supervisory relationship. An interval longer than four weeks is questionable.

4 **Recording sessions**
This should depend on what the practice nurse wants. There is already so much paperwork to be dealt with in GP practices.

5 **Links with individual performance review**
This would need to be negotiated locally. GPs might appreciate the link between clinical supervision and efficiency and standards.

6   **Contract between supervisor and supervisee**
    This would have to be negotiated and agreed. It is very important
    to have a contract.

7   **Training for supervisor**
    Currently trying to identify a number of demonstration practices
    where practice nurses would have undergone relevant diploma or
    degree level work, who could develop some training. This would
    probably be in a group training practice.

8   **Supervision for supervisor**
    Supervisors must receive supervision. It may be that the supervisor
    would want supervision from a specialist in a specific area of prac-
    tice – diabetes or asthma, for example – and this arrangement
    could continue on a short-term basis – three to six months, say –
    when the supervisor would change to supervision in another area
    of specialist practice.

9   **Evaluation**
    This is crucial. Tools are available for measuring effectiveness of
    teamwork, and these might be appropriate. Areas to examine would
    include understanding of roles, job satisfaction, and so forth.

10 **Impact of clinical supervision**
    At the moment most of what we know is hypothetical, but the
    understanding is that it is very positive and refreshing.

11 **Place in business plan**
    All of this would have to be explained very carefully to GPs, clarify-
    ing the purpose of clinical supervision, and explaining the language.

12 **Additional comment**
    There will need to be a diversity of models. The work of the prac-
    tice nurse is very generic.
       A multidisciplinary approach to clinical supervision involving all
    primary health care team nurses would increase the potential number
    of supervisors. Some arrangement and agreements should be sought
    with the local trust so that cover could be provided for a particular

practice while the practice nurse is taken out of the service for supervision. This would be a particular issue for single-handed GPs.

Newly-qualified practice nurses should probably have a mentorship scheme, with the mentor being a practice nurse. The more experienced practice nurses may be prepared to have a supervisor from district nursing or health visiting. If that were to happen then it should be a two-way process, with practice nurses as supervisors to other primary health care nurses. For some very specific issues a nurse from the same speciality would be required as supervisor. A flexible approach is essential.

It is still too early to evaluate practice. At the moment we would look at effectiveness on the basis of the practitioner's views of her own changes. This is, of course, subjective. It is important to evaluate the aim of supervision, and to set out objectives and work out ways of measurement.

Model six   **From the perspective of the supervisee (1)**

1   **Length of time clinical supervision has been implemented**
     About one year. It was initiated as part of a two-way process. Health visitors felt the need. It was discussed in staff meetings. Line managers were supportive. A senior manager believed that health visitors were autonomous and independent practitioners and did not support the idea of line managers accompanying practitioners to case conferences or court, but was not necessarily opposed to clinical supervision *per se*.

2   **Nursing specialties involved**
     Health visitors, district nurses, school nurses.

3   **How clinical supervision is practised**
     Families of concern are discussed on a one-to-one basis. The designated supervisor is the line manager.

4   **Frequency and length of sessions**
     Every three to four months. The door is still open in between, for staff to raise specific issues and concerns. The sessions may last a

whole morning or afternoon, or a whole day. This is not fixed, but as requested.

5   **Recording sessions**
Notes are made as each family is discussed, together with a plan of action to work with each family. The line manager/clinical supervisor keeps these records on separate file, not with the staff file. The practitioner makes her own record of the plan.

6   **Links with individual performance review**
There was some appraisal last year. It was a complete disaster; stressful and the cause of much heartache. There was a basic lack of understanding. No-one had explained how it was to happen, and no-one had attended what was described as the important study course. Appraisal was shelved until everyone had attended the study course. The plan now is that everyone must attend and the situation is more clear. The HVA was supportive here.

There could be a link between appraisal and clinical supervision. It might be acceptable if the supervisor and appraiser were the same individual. On the other hand, they could be different people.

7   **Contract between supervisor and supervisee**
None.

8   **Training for supervisor**
Formal training not known, although supervisors did get together to devise a way of doing what they are doing. The supervisor is a qualified health visitor with two years' experience.

9   **Supervision for supervisor**
Not known.

10   **Monitoring**
It just happens.

11   **Evaluation and audit**
Unsure.

12 **Impact of clinical supervision**

It has made a difference. It is helpful and supportive. It is good to be able to discuss ideas with someone else and have opportunity to see things from a different angle, as it is possible to get sucked into family dynamics.

At first it felt threatening and was stressful; anxiety-provoking. We were afraid that the supervisor would focus on what we had or had not done, and that we would be criticised. It doesn't feel like that now.

The personality of the supervisor can affect the stress factor. Have experienced both being talked down to, and talked to. The latter is preferable; more relaxed. It is like two people working together, as equals, each respecting the other. Perhaps the first supervisor felt threatened or inexperienced.

Supervision is very positive if handled properly. It should improve practice. It removes the strain a little. Some personal matters can be mentioned.

13 **Place in business plan**

It will be written into the business plan.

14 **Special staff support services**

A staff counsellor is available. There used to be staff support in the form of self-help groups in the past, but not at the moment. There is too much going on. There are regular staff meetings.

15 **Additional comment**

To have more frequent clinical supervision: ie. monthly, would be difficult in terms of time. The chances are something unexpected would crop up – it is difficult to predict what will happen – and the session would have to be cancelled anyway.

Model seven **From the perspective of the supervisor (1)**

1 **Length of time clinical supervision has been implemented**

We use a package called 'person-centred supervision', which only touches the surface of supervision in health visiting. We have used it for the past year.

2 **Nursing specialties involved**
Health visitors, who in turn supervise their staff nurse support workers and the nursery nurses who carry out delegated duties.

3 **How clinical supervision is practised**
The health visitor is sent a letter with guidelines. The senior clinical nurse manager is the supervisor. The whole day is given to this. Auditing and monitoring takes place in the morning. Three care plans from different families are audited, and two families are visited. The practitioner is observed for activity, teamwork, knowledge-base and organisation and planning. Both supervisee and supervisor sign the forms and make any additional comment. When we visit the home or clinic, we ask the mothers various questions to see how they experience the service. Then there is a working lunch, where a number of issues may be raised which we can pick up later in the appraisal part of the day.

The discussion centres mainly on child protection issues or families. The practitioner highlights issues s/he wants discussed. The supervisor is not directive. The practitioner has to do the problem-solving.

When moving on to appraisal, the practitioner indicates what s/he wants to do next year in terms of setting objectives, and identifying professional development and training needs. Courses must be entirely relevant to the job, and if we wish to go on a course we negotiate that with personnel.

The practitioner is provided with the trust's objectives, and those of the supervisor. We try to ensure the experience is not threatening. If we discover anything of concern in the morning, we do not proceed to appraisal but stop and look at the particular matter and continue with that.

4 **Frequency and length of sessions**
Once a year. If staff wish to come back and discuss further, they do. Otherwise we provide day-to-day supervision, and can be contacted via bleeps.

5   **Recording sessions**
    There is a complete set of forms, and both supervisee and supervisor keep a copy. Records are not kept on the practitioner's staff file.

6   **Links with individual performance review**
    There are none. It is appraisal only, which takes place in the second part of the day.

7   **Contract between supervisor and supervisee**
    The letter and forms are received in advance. Confidentiality is assured. In the event of anything untoward arising, or possibility of malpractice, the process would stop and the matter would be investigated and records examined.

8   **Training for supervisor**
    Nine and a half days over three to four weeks. Training services were bought in. We trained with social services colleagues in a multi-disciplinary session, and training was paid for by the area child protection committee.

9   **Supervision for supervisor**
    None. Individual performance review should be coming in, but there has been nothing for years. No-one has the time. There was an appraisal one year ago.

10 **Monitoring**
    Clinical supervision is written into the supervisor's objectives.

11 **Evaluation and audit**
    None.

12 **Impact of clinical supervision**
    From the supervisor's point of view, the service is being monitored. Less time is being wasted, and a specific amount of time is being committed to a practitioner. Someone acts up in place of the manager, and thus has the opportunity to gain experience for her own development.
       From the supervisee's point of view, they have the benefit of

individual attention, and can explore many issues including their own career development. Morale seems to have improved, and people indicate they are feeling better. The sickness rates have been high, and it is too early to say whether clinical supervision has made a difference here. There are lots of staff vacancies.

13   **Place in business plan**
Appraisal is considered in the community review. There is the possibility that the person-centred supervision is to be included in the purchaser child protection contract.

14   **Additional comment**
We ourselves expressed the need for clinical supervision, and broadened it out from child protection issues. We felt that in health visiting everything is linked to child protection issues and children in need. We hope to pilot a group supervision programme.

The personality of the supervisor is very important. It is possible for health visitors to talk about issues that are not normally talked about, and we can ask: 'How can we meet your needs?'

We would only see a new member of staff for person-centred supervision after six months, to give them time to settle in. The supervisor would not cancel for any other 'urgent' meeting; someone else would have to go. In one year, only one member of staff (the supervisee) has had to cancel, because of illness.

Model eight   **From the perspective of the supervisee (11)**

1   **Length of time supervision has been implemented**
One year.

2   **Nursing specialties involved**
Health visitors.

3   **How clinical supervision is practised**
Group session with the clinical specialist as leader/supervisor. We discuss as a group any relevant health visitor issues, or specific topics such as PREP or a caseload problem. An individual may present a

specific scenario and ask others for their input, views, is there a better approach with a particular client or family. It is a way of getting other views, so you can check out what you are doing. It is particularly useful if you have become submerged in a case and can't see a way out; others outside may be able to see it more clearly.

4   **Frequency and length of sessions**
Weekly, for one hour.

5   **Recording sessions**
The facilitator takes notes and these are sent to the line manager, but simply to demonstrate we are using the time productively. The supervisees don't get a copy. The managers are very supportive and they don't interfere. It is a useful way to forward and raise issues with management. We have an agenda of general health visiting issues to focus discussion if there are no specific issues arising from anyone's practice. The agenda is agreed a few months ahead.

6   **Links with individual performance review**
None.

7   **Contract between supervisor and supervisee**
None.

8   **Training of supervisor/facilitator**
Some training.

9   **Supervision for supervisor**
Not known.

10   **Monitoring**
Through the minutes.

11   **Evaluation**
A questionnaire was sent from the facilitator asking us how helpful or otherwise we found it and did we want to change it. We wanted to keep it as it was.

12 **Audit**
None.

13 **Impact of clinical supervision**
We are more together with each other; there is less isolation, more liaison and more trust. I regard it as a bonus. It is one place where we can get to know each other, and where we do not feel threatened by management. As the trust builds up it is possible to be more honest about bringing and presenting cases. It is possible too to see when someone is getting really stressed, and this may be raised, including the cause: eg. caseload numbers.

There has been no difference to practice yet, but it is possible to see the difference in those of us who work with fundholding GPs; there appears to be more flexibility in ways of working.

14 **Place in business plan**
I think it is in the plan.

15 **Special staff support services**
In the main, these are from each other. On the whole people would be too frightened to go to the occupational health department. We have a sickness policy here whereby anybody who has a certain number of days off sick has to go to OH. Stress may be picked up there. It's nice to have clinical supervision.

16 **Additional comment**
I would rather have clinical supervision than not. I wish I had been able to have it from the start, when I first qualified. Any support is helpful.

Model nine **From the perspective of the supervisor (11)**

1 **Length of time clinical supervision has been implemented**
Two years.

2 **Nursing specialties involved**
Health visitors; school nurses; to include district nurses and com-

munity psychiatric nurses across the trust as a whole.

3 **How clinical supervision is practised**

Formal supervision is on a one-to-one basis every three months. Informal supervision happens more frequently, and we can look at training and development needs and the career plan. We are also developing a model of group supervision looking at child protection issues. For school nurses, the formal supervision mostly focuses on child protection, looking at individual families, or specific issues which have arisen at school, other issues and ideas.

4 **Frequency and length of sessions**

Every three months, on a one-to-one basis.

5 **Recording sessions**

This has been something of a struggle. Originally an attempt was made to use a rather prescriptive model based on Benner,[6] but no-one could use it. Supervision for child protection is documented in the records. For general clinical supervision, there is a discussion document and the practitioner keeps her own record. This is the model we use across our locality.

6 **Links with individual performance review**

None. Clinical supervision and IPR should be quite separate. Something may arise in supervision when it is appropriate to formulate an objective. The trust is looking at setting team objectives.

7 **Contract between supervisor and supervisee**

None. There is informal discussion at the beginning. At the moment there is no choice of supervisor, but we are looking at that.

8 **Training of supervisor**

We have a responsibility to keep up-to-date, and we attended a full-day course developing a model of clinical supervision. The senior nurse, quality adviser was involved in this. In group work on the day we looked at what clinical supervision is and what it isn't, and the client, the supervisee, the supervisor, and the relationship between them.

9 **Supervision for the supervisor**
None at the moment. We hope to address this soon. There is informal peer group supervision/support.

10 **Monitoring**
Informal. Managers check out that it is happening. It is written into our own objectives and is explicit in the team leader role and is in our job description.

11 **Evaluation**
Too early.

12 **Audit**
Two people have been involved in doing research projects. They have looked at quality, expectations, change of practice, current levels of supervision, and at how often it is happening.

13 **Impact of clinical supervision**
It is time-consuming getting the system up and running. But as practitioners, staff feel more supported and clearer about their professional development; personally they feel clearer about their boundaries. There is a chance to off-load and share burdens.

14 **Additional comment**
There has to be some way of ensuring people have a way to reflect on practice that links with standards, quality, outcomes and audit; a chance to examine how effective the work is.

The practitioner can't be all things to all people. There has to be a realistic way of working, not working with unrealistic goals and therefore setting oneself up to fail. Practitioners need to be given permission to move away from traditional models and to respond creatively to needs.

There is a place in supervision for challenging; for getting the right balance. It ought to be possible for audit and monitoring to take place without people feeling threatened, but it has to be done in the right way and there is a lot of work to be done in getting this right. A lot depends on the individual supervisor's personality, skill, ability and credibility.

Model ten   **From the perspective of supervisor and supervisee**

1   **Length of time clinical supervision has been implemented**
One year to 18 months.

2   **Nursing specialties involved**
Health visitors, district nurses and specialist nurses (Macmillan nurses and nurses from the disabilities team). Not practice nurses, as they are employed by GPs.

3   **How clinical supervision is practised**
On a one-to-one basis, and looking at any issues the supervisee wishes to raise. We had difficulties at first finding a suitable venue – a quiet office with no phones ringing or people interrupting. That was in the early days. It's rare now.

The issues brought are often to do with families: difficult cases, the action taken. Clinical supervision is a form of reflective practice: what could I look at or do now; what should I have done? Sometimes there is nothing else that could have been done. The feedback might be that the right course of action has been taken. From time to time professional development issues arise.

4   **Frequency and length of session**
Weekly to monthly. No less frequent than once a month. Management suggested fortnightly, but we thought there was sufficient informal supervision for once a month to be enough. But you can have it more frequently.

5   **Recording sessions**
The procedure came from guidelines from the mental health directorate. Either party can note things down. The supervisee usually keeps the record, unless the supervisor want a copy as well. The supervisor would keep her copy in a plain envelope, in a secure place. The supervisee may keep hers at home, or somewhere safe.

6   **Links with individual performance review**
None. The managers at the IPR will ask if clinical supervision is happening; if we are finding it effective; if it is working for us. They

won't ask for any details; simply to know it is happening. It is not at all threatening when they ask.

7 **Contract between supervisor and supervisee**
This is when the ground rules are set about frequency, place, confidentiality, length of time, and other issues such as when confidentiality cannot continue – when there is bad practice, or if something is happening that is harmful to a client or staff member. We would hope that the supervisee herself takes these situations to her manager, and she could then discuss in clinical supervision what management had suggested. It could be that the supervisor might offer to accompany the supervisee to the meeting with management, if that would be supportive.

It is a written contract, and both parties sign it. If the relationship breaks down, the supervisee can opt out and choose another supervisor. There is no fear of reprisal. We have to be aware that there could be a problem.

8 **Training for supervisor**
There was a half-day training session with the mental health directorate, which looked at what clinical supervision is, why it is important, how to do it, record keeping, confidentiality, problem-solving, using role play, and the use of counselling skills. Then there were two general sessions for all the staff, where management was also involved. Staff were given further information and the opportunity to ask questions – about reviewing the system, whether staff were happy about it, records, storage and so forth. Most people are pleased with how it is and don't want to change it. But the discussion allowed people to get together to talk about it, and they felt better about it afterwards. Not all practitioners wanted it at first. They felt that as they hadn't had it before, why did they need it now?

9 **Supervision for supervisor**
This is exactly the same as for supervisees, in terms of frequency, contracts and so forth. I have peer supervision 'back to back': that is, I am also supervisor to my supervisor. It doesn't have to be like that, but we chose to do it that way. We have one and a half hours

between the two of us. We meet every four weeks, and more frequently if necessary.

10 **Monitoring**
The clinical leader is in touch with us, and we have a code for clinical supervision on the Comcare computer system. At the moment there is no other means of measuring, and no forms to fill in.

11 **Evaluation**
It is discussed, but there is no formal evaluation as yet. We are trying to establish a method of evaluation, and to thrash it out with our audit manager. We are at the thinking stage at the moment.

12 **Audit**
Not known.

13 **Impact of clinical supervision**
There has been a positive response. People aren't grumbling about it. Personal practice has improved, and some problems get sorted out in a different way.

14 **Place in business plan**
It was included in last year's business plan, and so probably will be included in our present one.

15 **Special staff support services**
We do have a staff counselling service. It is separate from anything else, and does get used.

16 **Additional comment**
We are very positive about clinical supervision. I think it's excellent. Newly-qualified health visitors expect it, and student health visitors are regarding it as a future positive thing – a permanent extension of preceptorship, in a way. Some colleges seem to be including it as an expectation for their students' future practice.

We also use clinical supervision with our nursery nurses. This had to be considered separately, as they haven't come along the same pathway as health visitors and are not used to reflective practice. Two health visitors supervise the nursery nurses, who all work in the same practice. The nurses had the choice to get supervision from health visitors at other practices, but they wanted their own health visitors, whose role develops as well.

Summary

Among those models found particularly helpful and referred to by contributing projects is the Bond and Holland development model of supervision,[4] the aims of which are 'to support, to inform, to be a catalyst, to challenge'. Other contributors cite Proctor's[3] definition of the 'formative, restorative, normative' essence of the supervision process as particularly useful.

Readers may also find relevant the work of Christine Byrne,[7] and her model for health visitor supervision in child protection work, which can be applied equally in work other than child protection. Child protection is, of course, extremely important and should be supervised by a specialist in child protection, but clinical supervision must in no way be limited to this area alone.

What is clear is that people in different areas will develop their own models and styles, and there may be different models in the same areas. A flexible approach is seen as essential, and willingness to seek alternative strategies if evaluation shows one way not to be successful. Certainly all the contributors are enthusiastic about the start of the process.

It is not appropriate to say whether one model is better than another; that is not the purpose of their presentation here. What matters is that a positive response is being made to the 'health needs' of the profession.

REFERENCES

1 Kohner N. *Clinical supervision in practice*. London: King's Fund Centre, 1994.
2 Association news. *Health visitor* 1995; 68, 8: 312.
3 In: Hawkins P, Shohet R. *Supervision in the helping professions*. Milton Keynes: Open University Press, 1989.
4 Bond M, Holland S. Developmental supervision in health visiting. *Health visitor* 1994; 67, 11: 392-393.
5 Butterworth C, Faugier J (eds). *Clinical supervision and mentorship in nursing*. London: Chapman Hall, 1992.
6 Benner P. *From novice to expert*. California: Addison Wesley Publishing, 1984.
7 Byrne C. Devising a model health visitor supervision process. *Health visitor* 1994; 67, 4: 195-198.

Conclusion

Clinical supervision will benefit the practitioner, the practice, the client and the wider community; the service as a whole and the organisation delivering it. Clinical supervision should be as important to purchasing authorities as it is to provider units. It will be cost-effective, and can be achieved without extra funding. It cannot be achieved without addressing the culture of the organisation and how time – and staff – are managed.

All these hypotheses remain to be tested; careful monitoring and evaluation are integral to the clinical supervision process.

The work of all nurses in the community – indeed, of all nurses, wherever they work – centres on human relationships and interpersonal communication. The quality of this will determine the effectiveness of the practitioner's practice. The fundamental emphases in clinical supervision are on the quality of the human encounter and the importance of human relationships; on what happens between people, and how an understanding of this can facilitate human development. There is no more important work than this.

Appendix 1

The British Association of Counselling code of ethics and practice for the supervision of counsellors

(Reproduced with kind permission of the British Association of Counselling.
Note: the Code will be subject to periodic updating and revision.
Contact the BAC for the most recent edition:
BAC, 1 Regent Place, Rugby CV21 2PJ ℘ 01788 550 899.)

A **Introduction**

A.1 The purpose of this code of ethics is to establish standards for supervisors in their super-vision work with counsellors,* and to inform and protect counsellors seeking supervision.

A.2 Ethical standards comprise such values as integrity, competence, confidentiality and responsibility.

A.3 This document should be seen in relation to the code of ethics and practice for coun-sellors. NB: the appropriate code to be used by those involved in the supervision of trainees is the code of ethics of practice for trainers.

A.4 Members of this association, in assenting to this code, accept their responsibilities to counsellors and their clients, their agencies, to colleagues, and this association.

A.5 There are various models of supervision. The code applies to all supervision arrangements. The code of ethics has three sections:

1   the nature of supervision
2   issues of responsibility
3   issues of competence.
     The code of practice has two sections:
1   the management of the supervision work
2   confidentiality.
     The appendix describes different models of supervision, and comments on issues that may be relevant to particular models.

B **Code of ethics**

B.1 **The nature of supervision**

1.1 The primary purpose of supervision is to ensure that the counsellor is addressing the

*   *In the context of this guidance, 'counsellor' should be understood to refer to the health visitor/community nurse supervisee.*

needs of the client.

1.2 Supervision is a formal collaborative process. The term 'supervision' encompasses a number of functions concerned with monitoring, developing, and supporting individuals in their counselling role. (This process is sometimes known as 'non-managerial supervision' or 'consultative support'.)

1.3 To this end supervision is concerned with:

a the relationship between counsellor and client, to enhance its therapeutic effectiveness

b monitoring and supporting the counsellor in the counselling role

c the relationship between the counsellor and the supervisor, in order to enable the counsellor to develop his/her professional identity through reflection on the work, in the context of this relationship, which will be both critical and supportive

d clarifying the relationships between counsellor, client, supervisor, and (if any) the organisation(s) involved

e ensuring that ethical standards are maintained throughout the counselling work.

1.4 Supervision is therefore not primarily concerned with:

a training

b personal counselling of the counsellor

c line management.

However, the skills associated with these activities are central to competent supervision.

1.5 The supervisory relationship must by its nature be confidential.

1.6 A counsellor should not work without regular supervision.

B.2 Issues of responsibility

2.1 Given that the primary purpose of supervision is to ensure that the counsellor is addressing the needs of the client:

a counsellors are responsible for their work with the client, and for presenting and exploring as honestly as possible that work with the supervisor

b supervisors are responsible for helping counsellors reflect critically upon that work.

It is important that both parties are able to work together effectively (see C.2.1 - C.2.4).

2.2 Supervisors are responsible with counsellors for ensuring that they make best use of the supervision time.

2.3 Supervisors and counsellors are both responsible for setting and maintaining clear boundaries between working relationships and friendships or other relationships, and making explicit the boundaries between supervision, consultancy, therapy and training.

2.4 Supervisors and counsellors must distinguish between supervising and counselling the counsellor. They would not normally expect to mix the two. On the rare occasions when the supervisor might engage in counselling with the counsellor, a clear contract must be negotiated, and any counselling done must not be at the expense of supervision time.

2.5 Supervisors are responsible for the observation of the principles embodied in this code of ethics and practice for the supervision of counsellors, and the code of ethics and practice for counsellors.

2.6 Supervisors must recognise the value and dignity of counsellors as people, irrespective of origin, status, sex, sexual orientation, age, belief or contribution to society.

2.7 Supervisors are responsible for encouraging and facilitating the self-development of others, whilst also establishing clear working agreements which indicate the responsibility of counsellors for their own continued learning and self-monitoring.

2.8 Both are responsible for regularly reviewing the effectiveness of the supervision arrangement, and considering when it is appropriate to change it.

2.9 Supervisors are responsible for ensuring that the satisfaction of their own needs is not dependent upon the supervisory relationship, and they should not exploit this relationship.

2.10 The supervisor and counsellor should both consider their respective legal liabilities to each other, the employing organisation, if any, and the client.

B.3 Issues of competence

3.1 Supervisors should continually seek ways of increasing their own professional development, including, wherever possible, specific training in the development of supervision skills.

3.2 Supervisors must monitor their supervision work and be prepared to account to their counsellors and colleagues for the work they do.

3.3 Supervisors must monitor the limits of their competence.

3.4 Supervisors are strongly encouraged to make arrangements for their own consultancy and support to help them evaluate their supervision work.

3.5 Supervisors have a responsibility to monitor and maintain their own effectiveness. There may be times when their personal resources are so depleted that they will need to seek help and/or withdraw from the practice of supervision, whether temporarily or permanently.

3.6 Counsellors should consider carefully the implications of choosing a supervisor who is not a practising counsellor. This applies especially to inexperienced counsellors.

C Code of practice

C.1 Introduction

This code of practice is intended to give more specific information and guidance regarding the implementation of the principles embodied in the code of ethics for the supervision of counsellors.

C.2 The management of the supervision work

In order to establish an effective supervision contract, the following points should be considered:

2.1 Supervisors should inform counsellors as appropriate about their own training, philosophy and theoretical approach, qualifications, and the methods they use.

2.2 Supervisors should be explicit regarding practical arrangements for supervision, paying particular regard to the length of contact time, the frequency of contact and the privacy of the venue.

2.3 Fees required should be arranged in advance.

2.4 Supervisors and counsellors should make explicit the expectations and requirements they have of each other, and each party should assess the value of working with the other.

2.5 Before embarking on a supervision contract, supervisors should ascertain what, if any, therapeutic or helping relationships the counsellor has had, or is currently engaged in. This is in order to establish any effect this may have on the counsellor's counselling work.

2.6 If, in the course of supervision, it appears that counselling or therapy would be beneficial to a counsellor, the supervisor should discuss the issue and, if appropriate, make a suitable referral to a third party or agency.

2.7 Supervisors should ensure that counsellors are given regular opportunities to discuss and evaluate their experiences of supervision.

2.8 Supervisors should regularly review how the counsellor engages in self-assessment and self-evaluation of their work.

2.9 Supervisors should ensure that counsellors understand the importance of further training experiences, and encourage the counsellor's professional development in this way.

2.10 Supervisors must ensure that counsellors are made aware of the distinction between counselling, accountability to management, consultancy, support, supervision and training.

2.11 Because there is a distinction between line management and counselling supervision, where a counsellor works in an organisation or agency, the lines of accountability and responsibility need to be clearly defined, between: counsellor/client; supervisor/counsellor, organisation/client; organisation/supervisor; organisation/counsellor, supervisor/client.

2.12 Supervisors who become aware of a conflict between their obligation to a counsellor and their obligation to an employing organisation will make explicit to the counsellor the nature of the loyalties and responsibilities involved.

2.13 Where personal disagreements cannot be resolved by discussion between supervisor and counsellor, the supervisor should consult with a fellow professional and, if appropriate, offer to refer the counsellor to another supervisor.

2.14 In addition to the routine self-monitoring of their work, supervisors are strongly encouraged to arrange for regular evaluation of their work by an appropriately experienced consultant.

2.15 Supervisors should, whenever possible, seek further training experience that is relevant to their supervision work.

2.16 Supervisors should take account of the limitations of their competence, and arrange consultations or referrals when appropriate.

c.3 Confidentiality

3.1 As a general principal, supervisors must maintain confidentiality with regard to information about counsellors or clients, with the exception cited in c.3.2, c.3.3 and c.3.4.

3.2 Supervisors must not reveal confidential information concerning counsellors or clients to any other person or through any public medium unless:

a it is clearly stated in the supervision contract that this is acceptable to both parties, or

b when the supervisor considers it is necessary to prevent serious emotional or physical damage to the client.

When the initial contract is being made, agreement about the people to whom a supervisor may speak must include the people on whom the supervisor relies for support, supervision or consultancy. There must also be clarity at this stage about the boundaries of confidentiality regarding people (other than the counsellor) to whom the supervisor may be accountable.

3.3 Confidentiality does not preclude the disclosure of confidential information relating to counsellors when relevant to the following:

a recommendations concerning counsellors for professional purposes

b pursuit of disciplinary action involving counsellors in matters pertaining to ethical standards.

3.4 Information about specific counsellors may only be used for publication in journals or meetings with the counsellor's permission, and with anonymity preserved when the counsellor so specifies.

3.5 Discussion by supervisors of counsellors with professional colleagues should be purposeful and not trivialising.

D Appendix

D.1 Models of supervision

1.1 There are different models of supervision. This appendix outlines the particular features of some of these models.

1.2 One-to-one: supervisor-counsellor. This involves a single supervisor providing supervision for one other counsellor, who is usually less experienced than themselves in counselling. This is still the most widely used method of supervision. Its long history means that most of the issues requiring the supervisor's and counsellor's consideration are well understood, and these are included within the code of practice above.

1.3 One-to-one: co-supervision. This involves two participants providing supervision for each other by alternating the roles of supervisor and counsellor. Typically, the time available for a supervision session is divided equally between them.

1.4 Group supervision with identified supervisor(s). There is a range of ways of providing this form of supervision. At one end of the spectrum the supervisor, acting as the leader, will take responsibility for apportioning the time between the counsellors, and then concentrating on the work of the individuals in turn. At the other end of the range, the counsellors will allocate supervision time between themselves, using the supervisor as a technical resource. There are many different ways of working between these two alternatives.

1.5 Peer group supervision. This takes place when three or more counsellors share the responsibility for providing each others' supervision within a group context. Typically, they will consider themselves to be of broadly equal status, training and/or experience.

1.6 Eclectic methods of supervision. Some counsellors use combinations of the above models for their supervision.

D.2 Points requiring additional consideration

2.1 Certain models require the consideration of some of the points listed below, that are additional to the contents of the code of practice.

Types of supervision (see below D.2)	Points for consideration								
	2	3	4	5	6	7	8	9	
DI.2 One-to-one: supervisor-counsellor	●								
DI.3 One-to-one: co-supervision	●	●	●	●					
DI.4 Group supervision with identified supervisor(s)	●	●	●	●	●				
DI.5 Peer group supervision	●	●	●	●			●	●	●
DI.6 Eclectic model	All relevant points								

2.2 All the points contained elsewhere within the code of practice should be considered.

2.3 Sufficient time must be allocated to each counsellor to ensure adequate supervision of the counselling work.

2.4 This method is unlikely to be suitable for newly-trained or inexperienced counsellors, because of the importance of supervisors being experienced in counselling.

2.5 Care needs to be taken to develop an atmosphere conducive to sharing, questioning and challenging each other's practice in a constructive way.

2.6 As well as having a background in counselling work, supervisors should have appropriate groupwork experience in order to facilitate this kind of group.

2.7 All the participants should have sufficient groupwork experience to be able to engage the group process in ways in which facilitate effective supervision.

2.8 Explicit consideration should be given to deciding who is responsible for providing the supervision, and how the task of supervision will be carried out.

2.9 It is desirable that these groups are visited from time to time by a consultant to observe the group process and monitor the quality of the supervision.

Appendix 11

Bibliography
Supervision of staff working with children and families

1   **Supervision**

Dearnley B. A plain man's guide to supervision – or new clothes for the emperor?
Journal of Social Work Practice 1985; 2, 1

Gardiner Derek. *The anatomy of supervision: developing learning and professional competence for social work students.* Milton Keynes: Open University Press, 1989

Hawkins P, Shohet R. *Supervision in the helping professions.* Milton Keynes: Open University Press, 1989

Kadushin A. *Supervision in social work.* New York: Columbia Press, 1976

Mattinson J. *The reflection process in casework supervision.* London: Tavistock Institute of Marital Studies, 1975 (reprinted 1992)

Mattinson J. The deadly equal triangle. In: *Change and renewal in psychodynamic social work: British and American developments in practice and education for services to families and children.* Massachusetts/London: Smith College School of Social Work/Group for the Advancement of Psychotherapy in Social Work, 1981

2   **Supervision in child care/child protection**

British Association of Social Workers. *Management of child abuse: guide, policy and practice.* See pp.60-62: Code of practice for the supervisors of social workers dealing with child abuse. Birmingham: BASW, 1988

Department of health. *Working with child sexual abuse: guidelines for trainers and managers in social services departments.* London: HMSO, 1991

Morrison T. The emotional effects of child protection work on the worker. *Practice* 1991; 4, 4: 253-271

National Institute of Social Work. Race equality unit. *Race in child protection: a code of practice by the Black and White Alliance.* London: NISW, 1991

Richards M, Paynes C. Staff supervision in child protection work. London: NISW, 1990

Sayers J. Talking about child protection: stress and supervision. *Practice* 1992; 5, 2: 121-137

Stone M. *Child protection work: a professional guide.* Birmingham: Venture Press, 1990

Waters J. *The supervision of child protection work.* Aldershot: Avebury, 1992

3   **Supervision in social work**

Atherton J. *Professional supervision in group care.* London: Tavistock Publications, 1986

Blech G. How to prevent 'burn out' of social workers. In: Martel S (ed). *Supervision and team support.* London: FSU/Bedford Square Press, 1981

Clare M. Supervision, role strain and social services departments. *British Journal of*

[85]

Social Work 1988; 18: 489-507

Cockburn J. *Team leaders and team managers in social services.* Social Work
    Monographs. Norwich: University of East Anglia, 1990

Coulshed V. Supervision and consultation. In: *Management in social work.* London:
    BASW/Macmillan, 1990

Nixon S. The need for working agreements: social workers' expectations of their team
    leaders in supervision. In: Cypher J (ed). *Team leadership in the social services.*
    Birmingham: BASW, 1982

Wandsworth Social Services Department. *Wandsworth's study and review of supervisory
    practice.* London: Wandsworth Borough Council, 1988

Wandsworth Social Services Department/Tavistock Institute of Marital Studies.
    Learning supervision. London: Wandsworth Borough Council, 1989

4   Organisational/institutional theory

De Board R. *The psychoanalysis of organisations.* See chapter 8: Human behaviour and
    general systems theory. London: Tavistock Publications, 1978

Kakabadse A. *Culture of the social services.* See part one. London: Gower, 1982

Mattinson J, Sinclair I. *Mate and stalemate.* See part five: The clients, the workers and
    the organisation. London: Tavistock Institute of Marital Studies/Tavistock
    Institute of Medical Psychology, 1979

Menzies-Lyth I, Isabel EP. A case study in the functioning of social systems as a
    defence against anxiety: a report on a study of the nursing service of a general hos-
    pital. In: *Containing anxiety in institutions. Selected essays volume one.* London: Free
    Association Books, 1988

Menzies-Lyth I, Isabel EP. Staff support systems: task and anti-task in adolescent insti-
    tutions. In: *Containing anxiety in institutions. Selected essays volume one.* London:
    Free Association Books, 1988

5   General

Britton R. Re-enactment as an unwitting professional response to family dynamics.
    In: Box S *et al* (eds). *Psychotherapy with families: an analytic approach.* London:
    Routledge and Kegan Paul, 1981

Colman W. In: *On call: the work of a telephone helpline for child abusers.* Aberdeen:
    Aberdeen University Press, 1989

Furniss T. Mutual influence and interlocking: professional family process in the treat-
    ment of child sexual abuse and incest. *Child Abuse and Neglect* 1983; 7: 207-223

Harkness D, Hensley H. Changing the focus of social work supervision: effects on
    client satisfaction and generalised contentment. *Social Work* 1991; 36: 6: 506-512

Marris P. *Loss and change.* See chapter one The conservative impulse, and chapter eight
    The management of change. London: Routledge and Kegan Paul, 1974

Pearson G, Treseder J, Yelloly M (eds). *Social work and the legacy of Freud: psychoanaly-
    sis and its uses.* See chapter four: Downes C. A psychodynamic approach to the
    work of an area team, and chapter eight: Bacon R. Countertransference in a case
    conference: resistance and rejection in work with abusing families and their chil-
    dren, and chapter nine: Simmonds J. Thinking about feelings in group care.

London: Macmillan Education, 1988

Pottage D, Evans M. *Work-based stress: prescription is not the cure.* Discussion paper number one. London: National Institute of Social Work, 1992

Schon DA. *The reflective practitioner: how professionals think in action.* See chapter five. London: Temple Smith, 1983

Will D, Baird D. An integrated approach to dysfunction in interprofessional systems. *Journal of Family Therapy* 1984; 6: 275-290

Woodhouse D, Pengelly P. *Anxiety and the dynamics of collaboration.* Aberdeen: Aberdeen University Press, 1991